God in Fragments

God in Fragments

*Worshipping with Those Living
with Dementia*

Robert Atwell
Joanna Collicutt
Matthew Salisbury
Julia Burton-Jones
David Richardson
Sue Moore
Sam Wells

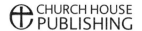 CHURCH HOUSE
PUBLISHING

Church House Publishing
Church House
Great Smith Street
London SW1P 3AZ

Published in 2020 by Church House Publishing

978 0 7151 2367 6

Typeset by Regent Typesetting
Printed and bound in England by
CPI Group (UK) Ltd

Contents

Contributors   ix

1 God in Fragments: Worshipping with Those Living
   with Dementia   1
   Robert Atwell

2 Spiritual Awareness and Dementia   14
   Joanna Collicutt

3 A Theology of Worshipping with Dementia   37
   Matthew Salisbury

4 Creating Dementia-friendly Worship   60
   Julia Burton-Jones

5 Dementia-friendly Churches   86
   David Richardson

6 Music and Dementia: Some Practical Considerations 111
   Sue Moore

Afterword   118
   Sam Wells

Summary of Advice and Recommendations   121

*Further Reading, Websites, and Bibliography for
Individual Chapters*   125

Index   133

In you, O Lord, I take refuge;
  let me never be put to shame.

Be to me a rock of refuge,
a strong fortress,
to save me,
for you are my rock and my fortress.

For you, O Lord, are my hope,
my trust, O Lord, from my youth.

Upon you I have leaned from my birth;
it was you who took me from my mother's womb.
My praise is continually of you.

O God, from my youth you have taught me,
and I still proclaim your wondrous deeds.
So even to old age and grey hairs,
O God, do not forsake me,
until I proclaim your might to all the generations to come.

(Verses from Psalm 71)

Contributors

The Right Reverend Robert Atwell is Bishop of Exeter and Chair of the Liturgical Commission.

The Revd Canon Dr Joanna Collicutt is Karl Jaspers Lecturer in Psychology and Spirituality at Ripon College Cuddesdon. She has written several books on psychology and faith including *Thinking of You: a resource for the spiritual care of people with dementia.*

Dr Matthew Salisbury is National Liturgy and Worship Adviser of the Church of England and teaches in the University of Oxford where he is Assistant Chaplain at Worcester College.

Julia Burton-Jones is Anna Chaplaincy lead and dementia specialist for the dioceses of Rochester and Canterbury, and part of a national working group developing Anna Chaplaincy across the UK with the Bible Reading Fellowship.

David Richardson is Vice President of Churches Together in Cumbria and Reader at Kendal Parish Church, and a former trustee of Alzheimer's Society.

Sue Moore combines her role as Secretary of the Liturgical Commission with work for her local RSCM Area Committee and directing a growing parish church choir in South East London.

GOD IN FRAGMENTS

The Revd Dr Samuel Wells is Vicar of St Martin-in-the-Fields and Visiting Professor of Christian Ethics at King's College London.

God in Fragments:
Worshipping with Those Living
with Dementia

THE RT REVD ROBERT ATWELL
Chair of the Liturgical Commission

With an ageing population and the average age of our congregations continuing to rise, the importance of creating worship
that is accessible to those living with dementia has shot up the
liturgical agenda. Rarely a week passes these days without an
article appearing in the press about research into the causes
and impact of dementia, the work of memory cafés, or the
promotion of dementia-friendly churches and communities.
Meanwhile, the word 'Alzheimer's' has become a byword for
fear and anxiety. Studies show that many people now fear the
onset of dementia more than they do cancer.

What does the Christian gospel have to say to a society that
lives in fear of dementia? This was the question posed at the
outset of a conference held by the Liturgical Commission in
April 2017 to resource those engaged in creating accessible
worship for people living with dementia. As well as being
topical, the subject is central to the values of the gospel because
in our ministry among people living with dementia we have a
unique opportunity to witness to human dignity in an age that
idolizes the young and the beautiful, often at the expense of
older people in the community. Words from Leviticus come
to mind: 'You shall rise before the aged, and defer to the old;
and you shall fear your God' (Leviticus 19.32). It is a sad

commentary on our society that buses and trains nowadays have to display notices encouraging people to give up their seat for an older person, as if this were not self-evident. The conference drew upon the insights and expertise of theologians, psychologists, musicians, liturgists and practitioners. We debated contested areas of theology such as the meaning of personhood when memory disintegrates. We explored the style, structure and content of worship best suited to those whose cognitive ability is impaired. How does liturgy work when the relationship between words and cognition is disturbed? What is its purpose and function? Of what value are the sacraments, including anointing? How do we pray with those whose sense of God and of themselves is at best fragmentary? How do we nourish their spirituality?

The conference was a day for comparing notes and sharing experience in an attempt to distil wisdom that can be shared across the Church in the knowledge that society is deeply afraid of dementia. This volume brings together some of the fruits of the consultation, together with a compendium of resources and suggestions for further reading. It does not venture into the medical realm or claim to be an exhaustive study, but is offered as a contribution to current thinking with a view to informing the Church's liturgical and pastoral practice.

Dementia and diminishment

Visiting my parents shortly before they died, my father appeared at the front door wearing his overcoat, wellington boots and a tea-cosy. When I pointed to the tea-cosy on his head he said, 'I know. It's cold.' I was embarrassed at his appearance, particularly when I discovered that he had gone up to the local shops to buy a pint of milk looking like that, but in the end did it matter? Things were complicated by the fact that my father was my mother's main carer. She was crippled with arthritis and housebound, but she did have her marbles, whereas my father had lost most of his. In the kitchen were instructions written by my sister, Blu-tacked to the wall, telling my father how to make a cup of tea. He could no longer remember. Nor could he remember how to shave. I used to tell him that designer stubble was all the rage, though not so fashionable when sporting a tea-cosy on your head. One day while shaving my father, he said, 'That it should come to this. I never thought my own son would end up shaving me.' This was the same man who had been a Spitfire pilot in the war, an accountant by profession, and the loving father of our family.

Just as every person living with dementia has their own story to tell, so every family accumulates a litany of anecdotes about their elderly, confused relatives. Some stories are amusing, others painful, some tragic. Many know at first hand the burden of caring for those with dementia and the guilt that can overtake you when patience finally runs out and you lose your rag. Crafting accessible worship for people living with dementia touches deep places where all of us are vulnerable. It is an art form, a hit-and-miss affair requiring basic practical know-how as much as liturgical expertise. It is challenging and also deeply rewarding as one watches individuals who ordinarily may be heavily introverted suddenly emerge into the light. Above all, it is rarely grim as those haunted by their fear of dementia often suppose. W. B. Yeats's poem about old age, 'Lapis Lazuli', speaks of the gift of years:

> Gaiety transfiguring all that dread . . .
> Their eyes mid many wrinkles, their eyes
> Their ancient, glittering eyes, are gay.[1]

There are thousands of such older people, including some with dementia, whose eyes glitter gaily amid their wrinkles.

Humour invariably breaks through in the best orchestrated worship. Visiting a residential home specializing in the care of people with advanced dementia, I was invited to lead an act of worship for some of the residents. The assembled residents were introduced to me by name, including Audrey whose preferred seat was next to the aquarium. 'You like sitting there,

---

1 W. B. Yeats, 'Lapis Lazuli', in *The Collected Poems of W. B. Yeats*, London: Macmillan, 1989.

don't you?' said the care assistant in an affirming voice. 'Yes', said Audrey. 'Fish are better than men. They're prettier and they don't answer back.' It was her only contribution to the proceedings but it broke the ice.

Understanding dementia

According to the government figures, there are currently 850,000 people living with dementia in the UK. It is estimated that this number is set to rise significantly over the next 25 years, with one in three people in the population over the age of 65 developing the condition. That person could be sitting next to you in church or it could be you. Dementia's age profile suggests that it affects mainly people aged between 70 and 90, but in reality it is not exclusively a disease of the elderly. When I was a student, the wife of one of my tutors developed dementia when she was only 45. We need to be wary of stereotyping.

Alzheimer's disease is the most common type of dementia and the one most usually spoken about, often erroneously. But there are other forms of the disease: vascular dementia, fronto-temporal dementia, and dementia with Lewy bodies, each of which exhibits different pathologies. Diagnosing dementia and tracking its progress requires specialist medical knowledge that lies beyond the scope of this volume. Nevertheless, as we attempt to devise worship that is readily accessible for those living with dementia it is important to be informed about the complexity of this medical condition and be alert to different patterns of behaviour for which allowance needs to be made.

'Dementia' is an umbrella term that embraces a wide variety of symptoms ranging from agitation, memory loss, confusion, difficulty with language and decision-making, to (as in my father's case) an inability to make a cup of tea. Changes in a person's behaviour may be small to the point of insignificance at first, but cumulatively they can become severe enough to affect a person's daily life and their ability to live independently. Restlessness, aggression, poor concentration, and inappropriate interjections in a conversation can all feature. Visual-spatial awareness can be affected. A person may no longer be able to judge distances easily or negotiate a flight of stairs.

In the early stages of the disease those living with dementia often feel cut off and isolated. It is not uncommon to hear reports of people being patronized, ridiculed or simply ignored. The worship we facilitate, therefore, must not only be accessible and allow people to participate to the best of their ability; it must enable them to *feel* included. This is important not just pastorally and psychologically, but theologically. The Church is the Body of Christ, a community of belonging in which, as St Paul insists, each of us has a valued place (1 Corinthians 12). The strong need the weak just as much as the weak need the strong. In a culture that often judges a person's value by what they do and their usefulness to society, the valuing of individuals for their own sake, as women and men made in the image of God and in whom God delights (Genesis 1.26–31), is itself a profound witness. In an increasingly materialist world we need to resist everything that dehumanizes or trivializes people. We should never underestimate how the values of our prevailing culture can infiltrate and reshape the life of the worshipping community.

In spite of considerable medical advances, dementia remains a one-way street, a progressive disease whose impact can in certain cases be slowed, but not as yet arrested or reversed. How quickly it progresses will vary from individual to individual and correspond to the type of dementia a person has. As the condition progresses, it can generate bouts of intense anxiety, introversion and depression. In spite of this, many manage to maintain their independence for several years with the help and support of friends, family and neighbours. Their presence adds another dimension to the task in hand because any act of worship we devise needs to embrace carers too and address their religious and spiritual needs. After all, they are experiencing the impact of this disease at close quarters as well. They are not detached bystanders, casually observing the progress of a degenerative medical condition. In their own way they too are living with dementia and, as a result, are often deeply emotionally involved. Coping with confused friends and relatives can be exhausting and distressing. People they have known for years suddenly no longer know who they are. Family and friends will bring their exhaustion and anxiety to any worship we facilitate as well as their love for the individual concerned. They yearn to be connected spiritually with those they care for, particularly when distressing symptoms proliferate and they watch the person they love disappear into a fog of confusion from which they know they will never return. In the words of Psalm 88, they become lost in 'the land of forgetfulness'.

When memory fragments

Dubbed the father of modern Western philosophy, the seventeenth-century French philosopher and mathematician Descartes is remembered for his statement *cogito ergo sum* – 'I think; therefore I am.' His remark has become a touchstone of Western thinking. As a result, rationality, memory and intellect are given inordinate importance as hallmarks of our humanity. But what happens when I can no longer think clearly? In a twenty-first-century variant on Descartes, we might also say, 'I choose; therefore I have significance.' Contemporary Western society has certainly exalted the virtue of choice to an almost iconic status. Many now see choice as an end in itself and the key to happiness and self-fulfilment. But what if I am no longer in a position to choose? Do I still have value in a scheme of things that seems to value productivity and achievement above all else?

Philosophy aside, biologists tell us that the ability to remember the past and to envision the future is one of the things that distinguishes humankind from the rest of the animal kingdom. I sometimes picture myself with a giant carpet-bag of memories inside me. As I journey through life I collect more and more experiences along the way. Some I discard and forget; others remain vibrant at the front of my consciousness. When I stop and reflect I find myself rummaging through my memories, often finding all sorts of unexpected things lying forgotten at the bottom of the bag. But what happens if my internal carpet-bag has moths and developed holes? What then? What happens when, as a result, I lose precious memories that chart my journey so that I no longer have a sense of the story of my life?

Memories infused with gratitude are undoubtedly the wonderful consolation of old age. It is why as we grow older the prayer of reminiscence becomes such a prominent feature of our spirituality, enabling us to savour people and events that have shaped us for good. Of course, when we pray in this way we can also find the experience disturbing. We find ourselves mourning friends we have lost or who have died, opportunities we squandered or mistakes we made. It is why being alongside people as they try to access and explore their memories demands real sensitivity. In our memory we meet ourselves. Helping those living with dementia to pray with their memories and their fragmented sense of God can be particularly challenging because their minds are jumbled and their memories often play tricks on them, causing them distress.

St Augustine likens memory to a royal court full of people: some familiar, others strange; some delightful, others threatening and disturbing. 'In the vast hall of my memory,' he says, 'I meet myself and recall what I am, what I have done, and when and where and how I was affected when I did it.'[2] In our memories we do indeed meet ourselves: who we were and who we have become.

The visit of a prospective MP to a residential care home in his constituency during the run-up to a general election has become legendary. Competing with the noise of the television, the politician knelt down on one knee to speak to a resident. Full of self-importance, he asked the lady in a loud, patronizing voice, 'Do-you-know-who-I-am?' The puzzled resident replied, 'No, I don't. But if you go to reception, I'm sure you'll find someone who will tell you.'

Memory is the matrix of our identity, which is why the onset of dementia is so terrifying. When someone no longer has access to the narrative of their life, we experience them

---

2 Augustine, *Confessions*, X, 8.

as losing their personhood and we grieve for them. When our memory fragments, the self is lost and with it our sense of God. We no longer know who others are or who we are or who God is. As the wife of a former colleague of mine said of her husband, 'The lights are on, but there's no one at home.' But is this true? Has the person gone? This is what we observe and fear, but is it true?

Personhood and the loss of memory

What does it mean to be a person? The onset of dementia raises this theological question with a degree of sharpness. If we define personhood simply in relation to our capacity for rationality or productivity, then we are in grave danger of reducing humanity to a cypher for functionality. The fact that a person is no longer able to remember the past clearly and therefore finds it difficult or impossible to envision the future, construct rational plans or make moral choices does not mean that they have ceased to be a person any more than an infant at the breast (who can also do none of these things) is not to be regarded and valued as a person. Personhood is not defined by cognitive ability.

Scripture is rich in images for understanding and honouring the enduring human person. As we have already noted, Scripture teaches us that we are made in the image of God. In the opening chapter of Genesis we read: 'God created humankind in his image, in the image of God he created them; male and female he created them' (Genesis 1.27). This is often interpreted, not incorrectly, as meaning that each of us is uniquely loved and cherished by God our Creator. But as the text makes clear, the image of God in humankind is one of community: male and female he created them. This is a richer seam for self-understanding than the individualism that dominates much of current Western thinking.

This theological understanding coheres with the realization that we are the product not simply of our DNA, but of the community in which we are nurtured and our environment.

Personhood is forged through a network of relationships. The family into which we are born, the community in which we live and relate to, all help shape us for good and ill. We do not cease to be a person just because we have lost our memory. Whether we are aware of it or not, we still belong, we are still part of the human family. And although we may no longer be able to safeguard our own memories, the community holds memories of us and, to a degree, for us. So does God. God does not forget.

'Can a woman forget her nursing-child, or show no compassion for the child of her womb? Even these may forget, yet I will not forget you. See, I have inscribed you on the palms of my hands' (Isaiah 49.15–16). Each of us is held unconditionally in the loving embrace of God. God remembers us even when we don't remember him. God knows us and calls us by name, even when we forget our own.

Crafting accessible worship

As will become clear from the various contributions to this book, designing worship for people living with dementia is an art-form. We talk about 'coming to our senses' but seldom think how this translates in the realm of worship. Using all our senses gives a richer experience to worship and aids participation. Sensory prompts can help access long-term memories. Visual images, for example, can be very powerful. Photographs of friends and family, icons, pictures of Jesus or of the saints, flowers, candles, can help create a secure and warm environment in which the prayer of reminiscence can flow. Praying with a simple holding cross in the palm of the hand can also help. The texture and shape of the cross may communicate where words alone will fail and be quickly forgotten. We do not know what happens to a person when they pray without understanding or how God is acting in this process. But Paul's words to the Church in Rome ring true: 'The Spirit helps us in our weakness; for we do not know how to pray as we ought, but that very Spirit intercedes with sighs too deep for words.

And God, who searches the heart, knows what is the mind of the Spirit, because the Spirit intercedes for the saints according to the will of God' (Romans 8.26–27).

When it comes to faith, research confirms that feelings remain long after facts have been forgotten. Liturgy is important because it enables a person to access feelings that otherwise might lie dormant. It offers a degree of spiritual freedom to those unable to exercise it in other parts of their lives. In liturgy repetition and familiarity stimulate engagement. For those in the early stages of dementia where they are midway between remembering and forgetting, but where language still has currency, using the Lord's Prayer in its traditional form, in combination with other familiar prayers, is immensely comforting. Reading from older versions of the Bible is also preferable to modern translations because it affirms identity and reassures people. As with all acts of worship, there need to be opportunities for thanksgiving and praise, for sorrow and lament, all offered to God in the hope of renewal, forgiveness and healing.

As with any service, the meeting and greeting of people sets the tone for what follows, as does the quality of personal preparation that those leading the worship bring to the occasion. The way a person stands, speaks, sings, moves and holds themselves will enhance or detract from the service. Good eye contact is important, as is the use of direct, clear language because ambiguity only exacerbates confusion. Periods of quiet for reflection are also important. Those living with dementia find extraneous noise and activity bewildering. Unsurprisingly, they also take longer to process what is being said or to follow what is happening. So pacing the act of worship in an unhurried way is vital if it is to be meaningful. It goes without saying that the virtues of patience, listening, simplicity and loving attention are writ large when it comes to leading worship with those living with dementia.

As language fades, using all the senses in worship generates a richer experience and strengthens a person's faith. If at all possible, carers should be involved in the planning of any worship, not least because they know those they care for well and can advise what will and will not work. Music often has a key part to play in 'unlocking the gates of memory'. To adapt the strapline of a famous advert, music reaches those parts of us that other things cannot reach. In this context the chapter on the role of music and hymnody is very insightful. Even when ordinary conversation is minimal, traditional hymns and songs that were sung in childhood, perhaps during school assemblies, can trigger memories in people and the words come flooding back releasing waves of reassurance. Music has the power to create connections. But it also raises profound missional questions for our generation about the function of liturgy and the place of music and song in worship, including the collective worship held in schools.

By and large, those living with dementia today were born between 1920 and 1940 at a time when levels of church-going in this country, although already in decline, were higher than they are now.[3] Mattins and Evensong from the Prayer Book formed the staple spiritual diet of most Anglicans. Learning psalms, collects and poetry by heart at Sunday school was usual. Every school, state-run or private, began the day with an act of Christian worship which introduced children to a modest repertoire of hymns from across the liturgical year. In old age those psalms, hymns and their melodies are still lodged in the minds of that generation. But what of us and the generation following us? Learning things by heart has gone out of fashion. What are we laying down in the memories of our children and grandchildren? What hymns will they know? Will the liturgy celebrated in our parish churches that they dip into, inhabit and unconsciously ingest nurture them in old age? What is the quality of the soul-food on offer?

Learning with and from those with dementia

The love and profound commitment that carers display for those living with dementia, often in very difficult circumstances, is a huge inspiration and has much to teach us, not least about

3 At present, 5 per cent of people diagnosed with dementia are under 65, and this number may rise.

the costliness of all pastoral ministry. Being alongside such people has taught me how precious God's gift of life is and the importance of attending to our inner selves. The older we get, the more fervently we need to pray that God will disinter resentment and heal our painful memories. We need to sort our relationships out before it's too late, and actively seek forgiveness and reconciliation for things we know we are responsible. None of us will experience the contentment at the end of our lives that God desires for us if we are not at peace with ourselves and our neighbour. We need here and now to keep our inner life true lest we wither inside and, in the emotive phrase of Joan Chittister, 'die from the outside in'.[4]

Over the years I have come to value a prayer for wholeness written by Evelyn Underhill:

O Lord, penetrate those murky corners
where we hide memories and tendencies
on which we do not care to look,
but which we will not disinter
and yield freely up to you,
that you may purify and transmute them:
the persistent buried grudge,
the half-acknowledged enmity
which is still smouldering;
the bitterness of that loss
we have not turned into sacrifice;
the private comfort we cling to;
the secret fear of failure which saps our initiative
and is really inverted pride;
the pessimism which is an insult to your joy, Lord;
we bring all these to you,
and we review them with shame and penitence
in your steadfast light.[5]

---

4 J. Chittister, *The Gift of Years*, London: Darton, Longman and Todd, 2008, p. 18.

5 E. Underhill, *Essential Writings*, Maryknoll, NY: Orbis Books, 2003.

The French theologian and philosopher Pierre Teilhard de Chardin found that praying in this way sharpened his hold on life and deepened his desire for God. Remarkably, he saw old age, illness, and even the prospect of increasing mental confusion, as opportunities to prepare him for the biggest adventure of all: the final surrender into the arms of God in death. He wrote:

> When the signs of age begin to mark my body (and still more when they touch my mind); when the illness that is to diminish me or carry me off strikes from without or is born within me; when the painful moment comes in which I suddenly awaken to the fact I am losing hold of myself and am absolutely passive within the hands of the great unknown forces that have formed me; in all those dark moments, O God, grant that I may understand that it is you (provided only my faith is strong enough) who are painfully parting the fibres of my being in order to penetrate to the very marrow of my substance and bear me away within yourself . . . Teach me to treat my death as an act of communion.[6]

In John's Gospel, following the feeding of the 5,000, we hear Jesus' instruction to his disciples: 'Gather up the fragments left over, so that nothing may be lost' (John 6.12). By the same token, though in this life we experience loss and diminishment, we believe that in the loving purposes of God, nothing will ultimately be lost. Indeed, God himself will gather up the fragments of our lives and memories and in Christ will make them whole.

---

6 P. Teilhard de Chardin, *Le Milieu Divin*, Paris, 1957; English translation, London: Collins & Sons, 1960, pp. 69–70.

2

Spiritual Awareness and Dementia

JOANNA COLLICUTT

In this chapter I consider the nature of human spiritual awareness, drawing on both the Christian tradition and insights from the psychology of religion, before exploring the many different ways that spiritual awareness may be affected by dementia. I go on to delineate some of the positive spiritual gains that can, unexpectedly, come with dementia, and set out some issues raised by the challenge of crafting meaningful worship for people living with dementia. Finally, I pose the question of what the future will hold as the old habits of liturgical practice all but vanish from our social fabric.

What is dementia?[1]

Dementia is a gradual, irreversible decline in mental abilities that is caused by an underlying health condition affecting the brain, such as Alzheimer's disease, Parkinson's disease, or heart and blood circulation problems. The nature of the underlying health condition determines the pattern and course of the decline in abilities; for example, in Alzheimer's disease the dementia typically begins with memory problems, but in other health conditions the first signs may be personality change,

---

1 For a fuller discussion of the issues in this section, see J. Collicutt, *Thinking of You: A Theological and Practical Resource for People Affected by Dementia*, Oxford: Bible Reading Fellowship, 2016, pp. 14–56.

speech and language, or the inability to carry out routine tasks such as getting dressed or setting the table. There is also a good deal of variation between individuals even if they share the same medical diagnosis, to the extent that in the world of dementia advocacy the phrase 'When you've met one person with dementia you've met one person with dementia' has become something of a mantra. While this rightly asserts the uniqueness of each affected individual, it should not deter the quest to draw out some general principles for understanding what people with dementia have in common.

Perhaps the most important of these principles is that dementia is as much a social as a medical condition. A diagnosis of dementia brings with it the prospect of long-term financial hardship related to care costs, vulnerability to abuse, social stigma, and isolation. The affected individual has a new place in the community or, sadly, often outside the community.

A second principle is that the affected individual is not an empty shell – someone who simply exists in a passive state as mental abilities are gradually stripped away, but an intelligent, active, and resourceful fully human being who does his or her best to make sense of what is happening. This will often be done by bringing a framework from the past to bear on the present (for example, a person with Alzheimer's disease may understand their care home as a boarding school) and then acting accordingly (waiting at the door for parents to come and take them home for the holidays). What may look irrational to the observer usually has its own internal logic. Communicating well with a person living with dementia rests on being able in some way to connect with this internal logic.

A third principle is that dementia brings a mix of losses and gains. The brain works by a delicate balance of many different systems that interact with one another. As one system goes into decline this doesn't show itself simply as a loss of certain abilities; the system may have worked by inhibiting other processes and, with its decline, these processes then have a freer rein. A simple example of this is what happens when a healthy individual consumes rather too much alcohol; the parts of the brain that exercise caution and discretion go into a temporary

15

decline, allowing increased confidence (good) but also giving aggressive or flirtatious impulses a freer rein (not so good).

In Alzheimer's disease the loss of rational word-based memory brings with it a greater emphasis on emotion-based memory, and the loss of recent memories brings with it a greater prominence of memories from the distant past. Examples in dementias arising from other conditions include the loss of the ability to attend to things on their left-hand side, bringing with it an excessive attentiveness to things on the right, or the loss of the ability to forward-plan – bringing with it an obsessive, pointless fiddling with objects in a quasi-purposeful way. Most notable of all, the loss of self-awareness and empathy that arise in some dementias brings with it inconsiderate, hostile or unwanted sexual behaviours. Dementia, at least in the early and middle phases, is therefore not all about loss but about a shift in balance; alongside the losses come gains that are often deeply troubling but that can sometimes be unexpectedly positive.

Recognizing the social and societal nature of dementia, the active logic that continues to work in affected individuals, and the mix of gains and losses involved is a prerequisite for building any approach to spiritual care of those involved.

What is spiritual awareness?

In the Christian tradition the human spirit is understood to be the part of us that responds to God and is thus the locus of a living relationship with God. This relationship is possible because we are, in some way, made in God's image; and this in its turn implies that relating to God has something to do with resemblance – that while God is 'other', God also feels deeply familiar.

The human spirit

The precise nature of the human spirit has been the subject of intense theological debate over the centuries, debate that is usually conducted within – and often constrained by – the fashionable philosophical conventions of its time. The New Testament is no exception, and operates with a number of half-stated anthropologies rooted in the thought of ancient Israel, but also influenced by the Hellenistic Judaism of its day, stretching them almost to breaking point in its attempts to make sense of the death and resurrection of Jesus.

The New Testament writers often draw a distinction between 'flesh' (*sarx*) and 'spirit' (*pneuma*). Theologically speaking, *sarx* refers to the values, goals and habits of this world that make people prone to sin; *pneuma* refers to the values, goals and habits of the kingdom made manifest in the Holy Spirit. But much confusion has surrounded this distinction because the Bible also uses *sarx* and *pneuma* in a simple biological sense (to mean 'fabric' and 'breath' respectively).

In an important passage setting out the theological meanings of *sarx* and *pneuma*, Paul links the Holy Spirit with its human counterpart and makes clear that the relationship between them is, as has already been noted, something to do with family resemblance:

> the mind that is set on the flesh is hostile to God; it does not submit to God's law – indeed it cannot, and those who are in the flesh cannot please God. But you are not in the flesh; you are in the Spirit, since the Spirit of God dwells in you . . . For all who are led by the Spirit of God are children of God. (Romans 8.7–9a, 14)

This theological understanding of flesh and spirit got rather lost as Christianity became influenced by Neo-platonist philosophies that understood human beings to be made up of two parts – a material body and an immaterial spirit. Theology became conflated with biology; for centuries the physical body and its material needs were understood to be essentially sinful, and the human spirit with its capacity to respond to God was understood to be ethereal and immaterial. This splitting of the human person was compounded by the seventeenth-century Enlightenment project, and in particular by René Descartes' separation of the material body and brain from the immaterial mind.

Yet the New Testament had always been more subtle and complex than this.[2] While it doesn't offer a fully systematic account, it seems to treat the human person as a unified body-brain (*sōma*) made up of a biological fabric (*sarx*) and animated by breath (*pneuma*); this is the substrate from which the personal human life functions (the *psuchē*) emerge. This life can be lived in an entirely worldly way (the life of the *sarx* in its theological sense); alternatively, something in the *psuchē* can respond to God by co-operating in a work of transformation. This 'something' is the human spirit (*pneuma* in its theological sense). Paul goes on to use *pneuma* in precisely this way as he continues the passage quoted above:

> When we cry, 'Abba! Father!' it is that very Spirit bearing witness with our spirit that we are children of God. (Romans 8.15b–16)

The human spirit is thus seen to be both relational and embodied. As Dallas Willard rightly asserts:

> Spirituality in human beings is not . . . a separate life running parallel to our bodily existence . . . It is rather a relationship of our embodied selves to God that has the natural and irrepressible effect of making us alive to the Kingdom of God here and now in the material world.[3]

It is important to keep in mind that theoretical questions about anthropology and epistemology were not the primary concern

2 For a full discussion, see J. Cooper, *Body, Soul, and Life Everlasting*, Grand Rapids, MI: Eerdmans, 1989; J. Green, *What About the Soul? Neuroscience and Christian Anthropology*, Nashville, TN: Abingdon Press, 2004; and M. Jeeves, *Minds, Brains, Souls and Gods*, Leicester: Inter-Varsity Press, 2013.

3 D. Willard, *The Spirit of the Disciplines: Understanding How God Changes Lives*, New York: HarperCollins, 1988, p. 31.

of the New Testament writers. Their agenda was pastoral. They were dealing with real-life concerns of flesh-and-blood believers who were facing bodily temptation, suffering and death, and who had pressing questions about what the good news of Jesus actually meant in these contexts.

For example, one of the most difficult passages in the New Testament arises in the context of unpacking the 'how' of Christian hope in the face of death. Paul argues that at death the *psuchē* shares the fate of the *sōma* that gave rise to it (though both live on in the memories of the community), but that the *pneuma* will rise with a new *sōma* at the resurrection:

> So it is with the resurrection of the dead. What is sown is perishable, what is raised is imperishable. It is sown in dishonour, it is raised in glory. It is sown in weakness, it is raised in power. It is sown a physical body [*sōma psuchikon*], it is raised a spiritual body [*sōma pneumatikon*]. If there is a physical body, there is also a spiritual body.
> (1 Corinthians 15.42–44)

Questions about resurrection continue to trouble us today,[4] but we also have a new concern: how are we to understand the spiritual life of those whose brains and personal lives have been ravaged by dementia? The 'natural body' spoken of by Paul is deeply damaged and, according to him, the 'spiritual body' is something for the future; so what about now?

The spirit's homing instinct

Christianity understands human spiritual awareness as embodied and about relationship but as also having a directional element, and that direction is upwards. Thus the New Testament tends to associate the life of the spirit with the world above or heaven: '"Blessed are you, Simon son of Jonah! For flesh [*sarx*] and blood has not revealed this to you, but my

---

4 V. Slater and J. Collicutt, 'Living Well in the End Times (LWET): a project to research and support churches' engagement with issues of death and dying', *Practical Theology* 11 (2018), pp. 176–88.

Father in heaven"' (Matthew 16.17); 'What is born of the flesh is flesh [*sarx*], and what is born of the Spirit is spirit [*pneuma*]. Do not be astonished that I said to you, "You must be born from above"' (John 3.6–7); 'So if you have been raised with Christ, seek the things that are above, where Christ is, seated at the right hand of God' (Colossians 3.1). There is a sense of travelling and, when this is combined with the sense of family resemblance touched on earlier, the whole can be aptly conceived as a return home.

Human faith is described as arising from a kind of homing instinct, the search of a child for his or her parent, by Paul in the speech on the Areopagus in Athens:

he himself gives to all mortals life and breath and all things. From one ancestor he made all nations to inhabit the whole earth, and he allotted the times of their existence and the boundaries of the places where they would live, so that they would search for God and perhaps grope for him and find him – though indeed he is not far from each one of us. For 'In him we live and move and have our being'; as even some of your own poets have said, 'For we too are his offspring.' (Acts 17.25b–28)

This is not too far from descriptions by social scientists who have moved from seeing human spirituality as a fixed ability or personality trait to a more dynamic quality of seeking[5] that involves self-transcendence.[6] The notion of transcendence suggests that we might supplement the idea of a 'homing instinct' with that of being stretched beyond one's habitual ways of being in the world.[7] This involves reaching beyond immediate con-

---

5 C. D. Batson, P. Schoenrade and W. L. Ventis, *Religion and the Individual: A Social-Psychological Perspective*, New York: Oxford University Press, 1993; K. Pargament, *The Psychology of Religion and Coping*, New York: Guilford, 2001.

6 P. Huguelet and H. Koenig, 'Introduction: key concepts', in P. Huguelet and H. Koenig (eds), *Religion and Spirituality in Psychiatry*, Cambridge: Cambridge University Press, 2009, pp. 1–5.

7 For a full description, see J. Collicutt, 'Posttraumatic growth, spirituality, and acquired brain injury', *Brain Impairment* 12 (2011a),

cerns to the ultimate or cosmic, reaching beyond self-interest to connect in empathy with others, and reaching beyond the chatter of mental thought into a place of inner stillness.

This homing instinct is sometimes awakened by a call or a memory (both beautifully depicted in William Holman Hunt's 1854 painting *The Awakening Conscience*[8]); it may show itself as attentive vigilance or active seeking. While social scientists remain agnostic on the ultimate origins of such awakenings, the Christian tradition understands this as a coming to life of the image of God with which all human beings are stamped; this happens as a response to signals of the divine in the natural world, human relationships, the creative arts; participation in worship; or reading the Bible.

The individual may be unsure whom or what he or she is seeking but the search will always involve identifying significance and making meaning. In neurotypical adults this shows itself as conscious engagement with the big questions of life, concerning its purpose, its benevolence, and the right way to live; and with big questions about the person, concerning identity and self-worth.[9] To this extent, spiritual awareness is dependent on a reasonable level of cognitive function.

How is spiritual awareness affected in dementia?

Losses in dementia

Human cognition is an aspect of the *psuchē* (or human psychology), which is in its turn brain-based.[10] In the previous section human spiritual awareness has been presented as arising from a homing instinct, awakened in response to

pp. 82–92, and 'Psychology, religion and spirituality', *The Psychologist* 24 (2011b), pp. 250–1.

8 Image at www.tate.org.uk/art/artworks/hunt-the-awakening-con science-t02075.

9 R. Baumeister, *Meanings of Life*, New York: Guilford, 1992.

10 J. Saver and J. Rabin, 'The neural substrates of religious experience', *Journal of Neuropsychiatry and Clinical Neuroscience* 9 (1997), pp. 498–510.

signals of transcendence, and involving a stretching beyond oneself, usually in the form of engagement with deep questions of meaning. Many of the psychological building blocks necessary to engage with such questions are affected by the brain changes that come with dementia, resulting in what I have termed elsewhere as 'transcendence deficits'.[11]

First, one needs rationality, language and memory to be able to frame and engage with deep questions of meaning and purpose, to pursue logical trains of thought, and to recall where you were in an argument. Healthy 'executive' functioning (being able to plan strategically, to generate a goal, keep that goal in mind, and to pursue it without becoming diverted) is particularly important here. It is also important in the making of moral judgements because it allows one to see things from more than one point of view. Impaired executive function is the hallmark of frontotemporal lobe dementia, but can also be seen in other types of dementia.

Memory also plays a part. It is not only necessary to keep one's train of thought ('working memory'), but also to refer back to facts and events from the past. Loss of 'autobiographical memory', as its name suggests, has a devastating effect on the ability to recall and tell one's life story. Hence engaging with questions of identity becomes very challenging, even to the extent of not being able to recall one's own name – a devastating loss. Memory impairment is the hallmark of Alzheimer's disease.

Language is also important in this regard. For some people (with vascular dementia or atypical Alzheimer's), speaking and thinking in words is no longer possible. Often these individuals have a relatively good memory, but without words their capacity for reflective thought is greatly impoverished, and of course they can no longer *tell* their stories.

Engagement with questions of self-worth may be impeded not so much by the health condition itself but by the social stigma it carries. People newly diagnosed with dementia are vulnerable to feelings of low self-worth and clinical depression,

---

11 Collicutt, 'Posttraumatic growth', p. 86.

and these may persist as the condition progresses. These in turn are likely to bring with them cognitive biases that skew self-appraisal in a negative direction, making it harder to hear and receive positive information, including information about one's human value. On top of that, the almost inevitable gradual withdrawal from social occasions removes one from access to the social capital available in the community, in the form of people who can help in navigating these issues by listening, affirming, challenging, or offering a broader perspective.

In dementia there is therefore a profound loss of the cognitive wherewithal to engage with big life questions (including the question of what it means to have dementia and why I have been 'unlucky' enough to get it). Furthermore, engaging with such questions in a way that stretches the boundaries, and moves one into a new place, is additionally challenging. For example, hope requires both memory for the past and the executive ability to imagine a future connected with where one is now but different from it (and thus to transcend the constrictions of one's immediate situation). Rowan Williams writes powerfully in his book called *Resurrection* about the threat to the very existence of the human spirit when such transcendence is no longer possible.[12]

Cognitive impairment also compromises the capacity to maintain rewarding relationships. For example, intact executive function enables one to see things from the other's point of view ('theory of mind'), and to transcend a perspective that is exclusively egocentric. Without empathy or a sense of solidarity, relationships flounder. Memory loss expressed in repeated questioning, the forgetting of loved ones (even longstanding partners and spouses), or the mistaking of grandchildren for children also takes its toll on relationships. And relationship is the stuff of spiritual life.

Finally, especially in the more advanced phases of dementia, the ability to be mentally and physically still, to meditate and

---

12 R. Williams, *Resurrection: Interpreting the Easter Gospel*, London: Darton, Longman and Todd, 2014, pp. 31–2.

pray, to transcend worry and anxiety through disciplining one's thought processes, may be lost.

In summary, dementia makes it hard to frame and engage with big questions and even harder to bring a transcendent dimension to the task; and it can erode relationships with the community that might otherwise be supportive. If the spiritual life is understood as a kind of journey home then the journey becomes one where the compass may be continually spinning, where recollection of the starting point has been lost, and through a landscape from which the usual signposts, markers and wise guides may have all but disappeared. But the homing instinct remains, the need for intimacy and connectedness is if anything stronger, and the result can then be not only a sense of disorientation, but one of alienation and abandonment.

Yet the reality evident to anyone who encounters people with dementia in more than the most superficial way is that their spiritual lives continue, though in different (and sometimes distressing) forms.

Positive gains in dementia

Earlier in this chapter the idea that dementia is a balance of losses and gains was introduced. The losses are unwanted and so are many of the gains. Nevertheless, there are some unexpected positive gains and insights that come with dementia, not only for the affected individuals and their loved ones but, if we are prepared to receive them, for society more broadly and for the Church in particular. One of the things to be learnt is that there are more ways of making meaning than explicitly engaging with propositions and questions by logical reasoning, or telling one's story in a verbal linear form:

> Contact with dementia . . . can – and indeed should – take us out of our customary patterns of over-busyness, hypercognitivism, and extreme talkativity, into a way of being in which emotion and feeling are given a much larger place. People who have dementia, for whom the life of emotions is often

intense, and without the ordinary forms of inhibition, may have something important to teach the rest of humankind.[13]

The shape and pattern of their stories will change. A person with dementia may no longer be able to construct a word-based continuous narrative either for themselves or to share with those around them, but there will still be a story. It will instead be expressed through basic habits, semi-preserved skills and gut feelings. The story won't be a coherent whole; it will be a series of flashbulb memories, of inchoate moods and fragments of purposeful behaviour.[14]

The fact that the spiritual life can continue for people who no longer have the cognitive wherewithal to do spirituality in the way we normally understand it should alert us to these alternative ways of meaning-making. It should also remind us that the spiritual life of those of us whose cognition is intact may be less dependent on the conventional forms of rationality and verbal propositional language than we might have assumed:

> I would want to argue for the importance in religious cognitive processing of the implicational system, a subsystem concerned with meanings, albeit at a non-propositional level. Indeed the discernment of such meanings seems to be at the heart of religion . . . It is not unusual for important but difficult insights to be glimpsed initially at the level of inarticulate meanings . . .[15]

It is as if deeper forms of making meaning (referred to as 'implicational' by Watts in the extract above) have been revealed, forms that are further back in our evolutionary history as a

---

13 T. Kitwood, *Dementia Reconsidered: The Person Comes First*, Maidenhead: Open University Press, 1997, p. 5.

14 J. Collicutt, *Thinking of You: A Theological and Practical Resource for People Affected by Dementia*, Oxford: Bible Reading Fellowship, 2016, p. 78.

15 F. Watts, *Theology and Psychology*, Aldershot: Ashgate, 2002, p. 87.

species and deeper in our subconscious as individuals. The reason for this is the pattern and course of brain impairment in dementia. In Alzheimer's the early damage is to the memory centres involved with 'explicit memory' – the ability consciously and intentionally to recall facts and events in an ordered fashion. In vascular dementia the whole cerebral cortex is compromised by a loss of blood supply; it would normally support a whole range of 'higher cognitive functions' involving knowledge and assumptions about the way the world is, and the representation of this knowledge in formal language. As already mentioned and as its name suggests, in frontotemporal dementia the early damage is to the frontal lobes, which support executive function. These are the last part of the brain to develop, not reaching full maturity until we are well into our twenties.

The general direction of travel in dementia is then to fall back on functions supported by other brain areas. These tend to be the subcortical centres that support different forms of memory and different ways of being in the world, forms and ways relied on by animals and very young children: learning to associate one thing with another rather than recalling events and facts; representing the world in terms of patterns of movement, action and the body rather than more abstract mental maps; relying on emotional hunches and intuition rather than rational argument; responding to the immediate sensory and aesthetic features (such as scent, colour and sounds) of a situation rather than its future implications; inhabiting language in terms of these sensory features and using it for emotional expression rather than instrumental communication. This shift in thinking modality transports the individual not just back to a previous way of being in the world but to the times when this thinking modality was operative, and so to the primal concerns of early childhood or the early days of parenting, and sometimes (sadly) to a traumatic time of life that was dominated by fear and other forms of emotional of mental processing.

This move to a more 'primitive' *psuchē* is on the face of it negative, and certainly represents a painful bereavement for all involved. But it also connects with Jesus' conversation with

Nicodemus about returning to the womb to be born again (John 3.3–4) and his teaching on the need to become like a child in order to receive the kingdom (Mark 10.15). Some of the gains that come with this move include less inhibition about truth-telling; greater freedom of emotional expression, playfulness and creativity; more poetic forms of speech that open up new horizons of meaning; a liberation to intimacy; and full engagement with the present moment (a feature of both mindfulness and the Christian contemplative tradition).

Two examples of this come from the stories of people living with dementia. The first was told me by a man whose father had never been able to talk about his wartime experiences for either reasons of social convention or emotional suppression. This meant that a significant part of his story was unknown to his family. As his dementia advanced, he lost this particular inhibition and was able to tell something of his experiences in those previously lost years. A much greater degree of intimacy and understanding with his family was achieved; in some sense he became more real to himself and to them, and this eased for them all the pain of his final days and death. The second story was told to me by a hospital chaplain who went regularly to the bedside of a woman with dementia on a general medical ward. She said short prayers, and when she ended with the Lord's Prayer the patient would join in. On one occasion when she arrived at the bed the family were gathered round it. She asked permission to pray with the patient as usual, moved close to her, and then began. When they got to the Lord's Prayer she became aware of sobbing behind her and, looking up, saw the whole family in tears. This was the first time they had heard their loved one's voice in several years; she could no longer speak but, as they discovered, she could pray.

This second story illustrates the familiar general observation that habits and routine practices laid down in early childhood and consolidated over a lifetime can be highly resistant to the onslaughts of dementia. We might think of this *habitus* as a resource on which to draw when other sources of meaning have fled. The spiritual care of people with dementia can then be seen not simply as a reactive process beginning after diagnosis of the condition, but one that needs to be attended to proactively across the lifespan by the intentional laying down of such resources, a point to which we will return at the end of the chapter.

There is then a sense that dementia, in stripping away some of our traditional methods for 'doing business with God', has the potential to take us to a place where it is easier for God to do business with us. We might think of this as a 'thin place'. A number of writers have suggested that these places are to be found not simply at sacred geographical sites or natural phenomena, but at points of human suffering, disability and disorientation – including advanced ageing and dementia.[16]

The fact that it is God who does business with us is a vital insight, easily forgotten when we feel masters of our own fate, but rediscovered in conditions such as dementia, where our dependence on our Creator is thrown into stark relief. Dementia has much to say to the Church about the grace of God, a topic explored at length in John Swinton's *Dementia: Living in the Memories of God*. As Paul points out in his speech to the Athenians quoted earlier, when we grope for God he is found to have 'not been far from each one of us', and as Augustine says in his *Confessions*, 'Late have I loved you . . . You were with me, and I was not with you.'[17] This should remind us of the Christian understanding that the homing instinct of the human spirit is not the only thing that leads us home; God's Spirit is at work in us, drawing us onwards (Philippians 2.13).

What is the role of worship in supporting spiritual awareness in people with dementia?

The notion of coming close to the God who would do business with us is the aim and rationale of Godly Play, an approach

---

16 P. Gomes, *The Good Book: Reading the Bible with Mind and Heart*, New York: Harper, 2002; J. Sorrell, 'Listening in thin places: ethics in the care of persons with Alzheimer's disease', *Advances in Nursing Science* 29 (2006), pp. 152–60.

17 Augustine, *Confessions*, X, 38.

described in some detail in Julia Burton-Jones' chapter in this book. Its founder, Jerome Berryman, presents it as 'about teaching the art of playing so one can come close to the Creator who comes close to us and even joins us when we are playing *at any age*'.[18] Godly Play is an approach to Christian spirituality that has its roots in the Montessori method of education and the form of Roman Catholic infant catechesis developed by Sofia Cavalletti.[19] It is highly liturgical in form: a Godly Play classroom is arranged to reflect the Christian story in accordance with the church liturgical year, placing the incarnation, represented by nativity figures, at its centre. Each Godly Play session follows the deep structure of the Eucharist: great care is taken in gathering and recognizing the space as sacred; there is a story told in word and action followed by a creative response from the participants; then there is a 'Feast' where a small amount of food is shared with reverence and attentiveness to the needs of all; finally, there is prayerful and orderly Dismissal. (Godly Play is examined more fully in Chapter 5.)

This deep liturgical structure is considered at least as important as the surface content of hearing a Bible story, engaging in creative activity, and eating together. It invites the questions of what is going on in a liturgical event and what its overall purpose is understood to be. Is it a form of therapy or way of promoting a sense of wellbeing in the human participants? Is it a vehicle for teaching and discipleship? Is it witness to the world? Is it an offering to God that in the process draws human beings closer to the Godhead?

The development of Godly Play illustrates this range of understandings and some of the ambiguities involved. It was originally conceived in the therapeutic environment of a paediatric hospital ward, and was then promoted as a form of religious education.[20] It has been framed as an 'evangelistic

---

18 J. Berryman, *Godly Play: An Imaginative Approach to Religious Education*, San Francisco, CA: Harper, 1991, p. 12; my italics.

19 S. Cavalletti, *The Religious Potential of the Child*, Chicago, IL: Archdiocese of Chicago, 1993.

20 Berryman, *Godly Play*, p. 12.

strategy';[21] used as worship in school assemblies; and more recently, presented as a method of spiritual formation across the whole lifespan.[22]

In his book *Pastoral Care in Worship: Liturgy and Psychology in Dialogue*, Neil Pembroke argues that while Christian liturgy may have a strongly pastoral – even therapeutic – aspect, it should never be defined by it, asserting that 'the only worship that is spiritually nourishing is that which is theocentric in orientation . . . the sacrifice of praise is the central act in worship; pastoral care is a support act'.[23] This – with the caveat that the central and support acts are not randomly connected but part of a greater coherent whole – is an apt caution against an overly instrumentalist anthropocentric approach to crafting liturgy for people with dementia. Nevertheless, it is precisely because liturgical worship engages with the embodied, emotive, intuitive, sensory and playful forms of being in the world and making meaning described in the previous section that it can be such a potent form of both spiritual formation and pastoral care for these people.

In the final part of this chapter I consider three ways in which liturgical worship can helpfully speak into the lives of people with dementia: by informing a theology of re-membering in the Eucharist; by enabling healthy lament; and by providing landmarks for the journey into this strange land.[24]

Re-membering in the Eucharist

The deep structure of Godly Play is eucharistic: gathering; word; sacred meal; dismissal. The central words 'Do this in remembrance of me' are not spoken, but instead enacted

21 M. Warner, 'Incarnation and church growth', in D. Goodhew (ed.), *Towards a Theology of Church Growth*, London: Routledge, 2015, pp. 107–26, 108.

22 www.godlyplay.uk/method/.

23 N. Pembroke, *Pastoral Care in Worship: Liturgy and Psychology in Dialogue*, London: T&T Clark, 2009, p. 2.

24 M. Goldsmith, *In a Strange Land . . .: People with Dementia and the Local Church*, Southwell: 4M Publications, 2004.

through this structure. Remembering is at the heart of the Eucharist and, if 'the tragedy of dementia is not so much that individuals forget as that they are forgotten',[25] then remembering is seen to be a sacred and pastoral act. This remembering is not only conscious and verbal; it involves ritual and symbol that both re-enacts a foundational event and reconstitutes the community. The body of Christ in that place is seen to be re-membered around the communion table, and as such the presence of Christ is made real, the community's identity is re-established, and it is resourced for its mission in the world.

This eucharistic structure is mirrored in the *psuchē* of the individual participant, and this is particularly significant for people with dementia whose mental lives have become unravelled and 'fractionated'.[26] There needs to be a re-gathering of what has become scattered; a reminder of the fundamental truth that all is well; a re-appropriation of the historical story on which that conviction is based; and a call to continue the journey in this light. All of this is signalled in the language and actions that are used in the Eucharist and, if we are alert to this, can fruitfully inform a pastoral agenda for people whose lives have become unravelled for any reason, including – but not limited to – dementia.

The words 'Gathering' (redolent of the fragments of bread and fish gathered up by the disciples after the feeding of the multitudes) and 'Collect' point to the task in hand. The Prayer of Preparation is a reminder that we are not forgotten by God and that the spiritual life is one of co-operation between the divine and human spirits. At the centre of the Liturgy of the Word is the proclamation of Good News. This central gospel message may often have to be opened and communicated without words to people in advanced stages of dementia. I once did this in a residential care home, communicating the deep structure of the Epiphany story simply by my tone of voice and bodily posture. I used knitted crib figures – the three wise

---

25 Collicutt, *Thinking of You*, p. 43.
26 A. Coles, 'The discipline of neurology', in A. Coles and J. Collicutt (eds), *Neurology and Religion*, Cambridge: Cambridge University Press, 2019.

men and the holy family – passing them around a circle for the residents, several in the advanced phase of dementia, to hold and examine. I then told a story of a long and arduous journey, walking around the room, dragging my feet, groaning in an exhausted and discouraged way, and then I picked up the baby figure and said the word 'joy!', clapping my hands and jumping. I then reflected (for those who had residual language) that this life can be long, hard and exhausting, especially in its final phase, but that at the end we meet Jesus and, like the Magi, we will be overwhelmed with joy. It was clear from the response that the group 'got' the message.

The Liturgy of the Sacrament is redolent with symbolic action and sacred speech. In the same care home there is a gentleman who regularly attends the service but does not receive the elements. He does not appear to know where he is or what is going on. He always wears a flat cap, even indoors; yet when I begin the eucharistic prayer he removes his cap. Something deep is calling to his deep.

For many others, the ingrained habitual response of holding up the hand to receive the elements is a reminder that bodily memory runs deep, and hunger for God comes before conscious memory and thought. The touching open-handedness is reminiscent of the child who asks his parent for bread (Matthew 7.9–10). This action of filial intimacy is a good theological and human instinct, for what follows receipt of communion (in the Book of Common Prayer, at least) is the Lord's Prayer (another bodily memory for that generation) said with confidence in the one to whom we bear such a striking family resemblance – our *Abba*.[27]

Finally, the Dismissal assures us of the continuing presence of God in our lives. It also reminds us that in the Eucharist we have been raised heavenwards to a new dignity, and that the call to live the Christian life 'on earth as it is in heaven' includes the call to live well with dementia. It thus communicates the hope that this is possible and reminds us that to be

27 For a reflection on Abba and dementia, see J. Collicutt, *When You Pray: Daily Bible Reflections on the Lord's Prayer*, Oxford: Bible Reading Fellowship, 2019, pp. 61–2.

fully human, and to have a place in the community, people with dementia must be able to contribute something. This last point may not so much require a change in their habits of giving as in our openness to receiving from them.

Enabling healthy lament

Dementia is a profoundly challenging condition because it forces us to confront more broadly the embodied and fragile nature of the human *psuchē*, and our mortality. We deal with our sense of disquiet and anxiety by investing emotionally or financially in finding better treatments and ultimately a cure, and by doing all we can to ensure that our loved ones are peaceful and contented. This is natural and understandable, and indeed the necessity of entering the inner world of affected individuals rather than trying to bring them back to the cold and unpleasant light of consensus reality has now become the foundation of best practice in dementia care.[28] Making people distressed for the sake of it is clearly wrong. Equally, the right of people with dementia to access treatment for coexisting mental health conditions such as depression and anxiety is increasingly being recognized.

But contentment all the time and at all costs is actually not a natural human condition. Our lives are made up of and enriched by a mix of losses and gains, of sadnesses and joys. It may be that our desire to remove all the negatives from the experience of people with dementia says something more about our anxieties than about their needs. There is such a thing as healthy lament, and the Church is replete with biblical and liturgical resources to support this. Mark Earey writes of the role of liturgy care coming from 'your "reality" being named'.[29] Exploring motifs such as journeying into the desert or dark places, of Sheol – the 'land of forgetfulness' of Psalm 88 – or of

---

28 See, for example, N. Feil, *The Validation Breakthrough: Simple Techniques for Communicating with People with Alzheimer's and Other Dementias*, Baltimore, MD: Health Professions Press, 2002.

29 M. Earey, *Worship that Cares*, London: SCM Press, 2012, p. 7.

being the lost sheep can be extremely useful in acknowledging the feelings of loss and lostness that are so hard to articulate adequately. Just as importantly, in connecting the individual's experience with the tradition he or she is reconnected with the community in new ways. Finally, the feelings are to some extent normalized and seen from a broader perspective. All of this applies to carers and family who are also 'living with dementia'.

The resources are there in specific texts, images, songs and prayers, but there is also again something about the deep structure of the Christian story centred on the Triduum that needs constant reiteration. This story does not avoid loss and lament; it is about a transformative journey through death into the deepest and most disorienting places of the earth before rising to new and unimaginably better life. Susan Marie Smith describes this motif, perhaps best exemplified in Psalm 22, as the 'critical criterion' for Christian liturgies that are truly pastoral.[30] People with dementia have a right to this sort of pastoral care and should not be confined to a diet of liturgical sedation.

Providing landmarks: what will be the 'Comfortable Words' for the next generation?

A recently ordained priest told me that he had come across the 'Comfortable Words' from the Book of Common Prayer for the first time when he began presiding at early morning Eucharists. He rather liked them and decided to include them in a sermon at the main service one day. He was surprised to see the older members of the congregation mouthing the words along with him, and reflected on the generation gap that this revealed. The words were new to him, but part of the fabric of these people's lives. He wondered what the equivalent of the Comfortable Words would be for his generation.

---

30 S. M. Smith, *Caring Liturgies: The Pastoral Power of Christian Ritual*, Minneapolis, MN: Fortress Press, 2012, p. 135.

Writing from the perspective of psychology of religion, Kenneth Pargament argues that religious ritual not only offers a way of making meaning at key transitional life points such as birth, marriage and death, by offering ways of transforming significance in these liminal situations (traditionally conceived as 'rites of passage'); it also provides the warp and weft or scaffolding within which meaning is held and significance conserved in settled periods of life.[31]

This sort of scaffolding, woven from familiar texts and the regular observance of certain practices, is the stuff of the deeper forms of meaning-making described in an earlier section, a kind of habitus that resources people for a lifelong spirituality. It has been available to Anglicans of previous generations through the words of the King James Bible and the Book of Common Prayer and, together with Shakespeare, has formed a kind of linguistic wallpaper providing the backdrop to our thinking and being in the world. This is crucially a *common* (though clearly not universal) backdrop, and as such it bound communities together (the literal meaning of 'religion'). This binding is not about producing rote repetition of uniform speech, but about provision of a shared poetic vocabulary within and from which people can do business with God and with one another, business that goes beyond words:

> Whatever else the Prayer Book stands for, the stability of its text has enabled people over time to internalise and make their own the words in which they worship God, in such a way that they enjoy a quite different sense of ownership of the liturgy than they can find in modern worship.[32]

31 K. Pargament, 'Religious methods of coping: sources for the conservation and transformation of significance', in E. Shafranske (ed.), *Religion and the Clinical Practice of Psychology*, Washington, DC: American Psychological Association, 1996, pp. 215–35.

32 P. Welsh, 'Time to retreat from throw-away liturgy', *Church Times*, 15 June 2018, www.churchtimes.co.uk/articles/2018/15-june/comment/opinion/time-to-retreat-from-throwaway-liturgy.

Its passing both mirrors and consolidates societal fragmentation. The prayers of individuals remain valid, but they no longer connect with others beyond their local worshipping community, if that. *Common Worship* is far too variegated and flexible in application to support this function, and it risks playing into an individualist clerical agenda.[33] The gathering and re-membering aspect of liturgical worship is effectively being lost in both a societal and an individual psychological sense, something that has been described as the slippage of a cultural and spiritual 'anchor'.[34]

We are where we are, and the world of the Book of Common Prayer cannot be replicated in today's more individualist, secular and multicultural Britain. But the fact that the next generation of people affected by dementia (within five to ten years) will not even know the Lord's Prayer should alert us to the need to review urgently the way liturgical worship might be used in new forms as a resource for individual spiritual equipping across the lifespan, and rediscover its capacity to bind the community of faith together with a common currency.

There is a general rule that what makes a community dementia-friendly makes that community more friendly to all. The needs of people living with dementia are very often the needs of us all experienced with particular clarity and intensity. As such, these individuals can be regarded as constituting a prophetic wing of the Church, and we would do well to attend to their voice.

---

33 Welsh, 'Time to retreat'.
34 I. Hands, 'Liturgy is an anchor – don't brush it aside', *Church Times*, 3 May 2019, www.churchtimes.co.uk/articles/2019/3-may/comment/opinion/liturgy-is-an-anchor-don-t-brush-it-aside.

3

A Theology of Worshipping
with Dementia

MATTHEW SALISBURY

I am who I am in the Body of Christ. (Christine Bryden)[1]

O God, from my youth you have taught me, and I still proclaim your wondrous deeds. So even to old age and grey
hairs, O God, do not forsake me, until I proclaim your might
to all the generations to come. (Psalm 71.17–18)

Much of this book is dedicated to advice about planning
and leading worship attended by people with dementia, and
addressing the many practical questions that worship leaders
may have about good practice and sensitivity. In this chapter,
I propose some ways in which worshipping alongside people
with dementia as equal partners in that enterprise contributes
to our shared journey as disciples of Christ and helps to build
up the Body of Christ, the Church.

There is great urgency in the task of shaping a Church
in which people with dementia are recognized, supported
and upheld, in an environment where many – if not most –
churches are themselves supported materially and practically
by older people, and where pastoral ministry to the elderly
occupies a significant amount of time. The ability to practise
one's religion is one of the top ten key quality of life indicators

---

1 C. Bryden, *Nothing About Us, Without Us*, London: Jessica Kingsley Publishers, 2015.

for people with dementia.[2] Most ministers, ordained and lay, quickly become involved in this work, and many are guided by their own experiences in which friends or family members have developed dementia. In particular, I wish to emphasize the substantive value of this approach, as well as the benefit of being with and listening to people with dementia themselves. Conversations about one's own relationships and experiences seem to be an immensely important and cathartic exercise, particularly for those who have themselves cared for loved ones. Such an enterprise of sharing one's experiences can contribute to a productive atmosphere of theological reflection. The sharing of anecdotes emphasizes the point that such experiences can and do happen to many people and, importantly, that every such experience may be different. Conversations about real experiences with dementia are also an important way of exploring the way Christians with dementia fit into the ecology of the Church. But discussions about worshipping with dementia, at least in the way they are recounted or analysed, fall in an awkward gap between the pastoral conversation and the often verbose – sometimes dispassionate – world of social science and psychology, and much of the scholarly literature (even if it purports to measure or describe accounts of spirituality) is insufficiently rooted in Christian pastoral response. Perhaps this is why some of the most helpful theological insights come not from empirical research, but rather from the experience of living and worshipping alongside, and ministering to, people with dementia, and most importantly from listening to their own voices.

This chapter argues that we need to take an approach to planning and executing worship that incorporates insights that are quite simple and essential: 1) that every case is different; 2) that we *all* engage differently with worship; and 3) that all Christians, whatever their particular characteristics or needs, are part of one body where they are together in God's love. While we need to take care that a person with dementia feels

---

2 E. Kennedy et al., 'Christian worship leaders' attitudes and observations of people with dementia', *Dementia* 13 (2014), pp. 586–97, p. 587.

as upheld in the structures and words of our worship as they can be, such efforts need to be incorporated within a much expanded and overhauled view of 'participation'. Competent vocalization is not the only viable sign of comprehension or spiritual benefit.

Listening to stories

The individual stories of people with dementia demonstrate not only the sensitivity that we must exercise given that every case is different, but also that people who look damaged and vulnerable are still living out the ministry of the baptized.

It is only too easy to categorize people with dementia as 'ill' or 'damaged' and thereby to dismiss their particular experiences as the consequences of a devastating condition from which it is not possible to recover; this can do untold violence to the integrity of a person's Christian life. In so doing we assume that a person with dementia, even early-stage dementia, has been damaged so much that they are not somehow who they originally were. We don't take this approach, on the whole, to people who are merely 'ageing' and who have lost some of the abilities they once had. The 'othering' of people with dementia, like most kinds of 'othering', may not be perpetrated deliberately, and people may be horrified at the thought of being at fault.[3] We affirm that all human beings are made in the image and likeness of God, but it is all too easy to suggest that dementia has damaged this likeness beyond repair. By that logic, it probably follows that dementia and other conditions that move away from the 'neurotypical' are seen only as an incurable and 'dreadful disease'.[4]

In fact, among the scholarly and pastoral discussions of the subject many commentators are quick to point out that what we call 'dementia' represents a range of symptoms rather than

---

3 'Other' as a verb stems from the language of sociology: in short, it refers to discriminating 'them' from 'us'.

4 M. Russell, 'Listening to dementia: a new paradigm for theology?', *Contact* 135 (2001), pp. 13–21, 15.

a 'disease' as such, which can be caused by a number of different pathologies – Alzheimer's disease among them. It is a state that can be reasonably compared to other kinds of cognitive dysfunction. Foremost among recent publications on the subject is John Swinton's book *Dementia: Living in the Memories of God*, which won the Michael Ramsey Prize in 2016. In the view of revisionist theologians and psychologists, dementia should be considered not so much an incapacitating condition afflicting the person that surpasses all the rest of their characteristics as individuals, but something that affects the way they perceive and interact with the people and things around them.

Some studies, citing the lack of quantitative, longitudinal data coming from the specific context of dementia, suggest that experiences of other kinds of cognitive difficulties should also be examined for helpful insights. The history of theological engagement with mental impairment or disability, for instance, is rather longer than its engagement with dementia. While it may not be pastorally helpful to compare someone who has been cognitively impaired from birth to someone who after a 'normal', long, healthy life has recently developed complex dementia, John Swinton and others argue that there is much to be gained from considering the literature and resources that offer ideas for worship with people with learning disabilities. Commentators often feel ashamed at the way that people respond to the behaviour of those with dementia or learning disabilities; while such behaviour is sometimes unsettling or unexpected, it is often met with disproportionate anxiety. Peter Kevern, among others, resists the tendency to think about disease, and points out that 'the one who disables also loses his humanity because he acts in an inhumane way'.[5]

It may well be thought insensitive to compare a gradually acquired, increasingly serious condition that usually attacks late in life to mental incapacity present since birth. But this possible insensitivity pales in comparison to some of the discourse that anonymizes a person's individual condition, and underlines

5 P. Kevern, 'The grace of foolishness: what Christians with dementia can bring to the churches', *Practical Theology* 2 (2009), pp. 205–18, 208.

the hopelessness and the inescapable end of the story. In the stereotypical understanding of dementia as terminal disease, described by theologian David Keck as 'deconstruction incarnate', there is no liberation but death.[6] The gradual loss of one's faculties implies that one loses a sense of personal agency, since conventional ideas of agency are dependent on 'control, thrift, rationality and success'.[7] As these traditional means of self-expression and engagement fail, it might follow that people with dementia become increasingly separated from the activities and relationships that they had previously invested with importance and that their experience of being a Christian becomes, in some significant way, impeded.[8] For instance, most theologians would assume that spiritual engagement is dependent on (in Swinton's words), 'an individuated, experiencing, cognitively able self, perceived as a reasoning, thinking, independent, decision-making being'.

Much that contradicts the view of Christian life as predicated upon rational intellect can be gained from personal stories, each about a unique and special person of God made in God's image and likeness, and indeed from experiences shared in the gathering of the Church, the Body of Christ. Memories of caring for someone whose own memory was unreliable are greatly valued by carers and ministers alike, and the need to share them may be part of a so-called 'talking cure' as much as it may be a method of sharing good practice. Telling stories about individuals also means that, by habit, people are not depersonalized into statistics or generic figures but, rather, retain their individuality even in their changed state. Anecdotes are given value by the authenticity of personal experience: this kind of learning through existing networks of trust is how we typically interact with people in our day-to-day relationships.

---

6 D. Keck, *Forgetting Whose We Are: Alzheimer's Disease and the Love of God*, Nashville, TN: Abingdon Press, 1996, p. 32.

7 Kevern, 'Grace of foolishness', p. 214; Russell, 'Listening to dementia', p. 15.

8 A. Phinney, 'Horizons of meaning in dementia: retained and shifting narratives', *Journal of Religion, Spirituality and Aging* 23 (2011), pp. 254–68, 254.

Sharing anecdotes may also be a means of validating or expressing solidarity with the experiences of others, and without a doubt certainly helps by expressing the widespread and complex challenges of dementia across geographic, religious and socioeconomic boundaries. It may also come from the wider context of 'person-centred' care which in theory now represents good practice in the NHS and for others who work with older people.

Placing emphasis on the particular experiences of individuals also helps to undermine one of the greatest fears of families, friends and, indeed, worship leaders: that dementia has erased the 'real' person from existence. What remains in this mythology is a shell that does not equate to that person's substance: they are 'already dead'. A deeply troubling but apparently popular poem, 'Alzheimer's', which starts with the line 'You didn't die just recently', may help to illustrate this view:

So we've already said, 'Goodbye'
To the person that we knew,
The person that we truly loved,
The person that *was* you.[9]

The narrator of this poem by Richard Underwood seems to be implying that the subject is in some way already dead; Joanna Collicutt, also reflecting on this poem, remarks on the fact that it presumes some sort of 'zombie-like' state.[10] While the conjecture that people who are actually present and breathing are not alive may be helpful for some, it seems rather discontinuous with a Christian understanding of the human person (to say nothing of the separation of mind and body). Complicating this reinterpretation of the faithful person with dementia yet further, some commentators consider whether a person is still a disciple of Jesus Christ if they have forgotten who Jesus

---

9 R. Underwood, 'Alzheimer's', available from https://richard-underwood.com/alzheimers/ [accessed 14 August 2019].

10 J. Collicutt, *Thinking of You: A Theological and Practical Resource for People Affected by Dementia*, Oxford: Bible Reading Fellowship, 2016.

is. Some people might even question whether someone with cognitive impairment can receive the authentic Word of God, or share knowingly in the sacrament of the body and blood of Christ. Yet Jesus Christ is present in their gathering, and especially in the sick and the suffering (cf. Matthew 25.31–46). Patricia Higgins writes of a 'dignity of identity' – that is, dignity rooted in the autonomy and integrity of the person. The 'real' person is still there. 'Even when you appear to have lost everything, faith will still be there, in the essence of you, like a perfume always remembered.'[11]

People with dementia do not have a monopoly on unfamiliar or unexpected habits in worship. 'Neurotypical' people have them too: the person with the tin ear who sings hymns lustily, the person who always stands at the back of the church, the person who insists on standing or kneeling when everyone else does the opposite. But these habits take on different significance when their root cause is regretted and feared. There is, of course, an argument that dementia, of one kind or another, may be intrinsic to ageing. The experience of cognitive impairment is also influenced by the way in which it is presented: John Swinton quotes an example from Stanley Hauerwas, who as a child encountered a woman whom he thought was his Sunday school teacher's assistant, but whom he later realized to be a person with Down's syndrome.[12] What do we gain from understanding that people with dementia are an inevitable and vulnerable part of the state of affairs of the contemporary Church?

The way to avoid the de-voicing of people with dementia (something that also happens within the 'theology of disability' and indeed in other areas of theological enquiry) is to listen to what the Spirit is saying to the churches through them. Stories are increasingly being told in the words of people with dementia themselves. At the time of writing, the BBC News website is playing a succession of videos of people in their

---

11 P. Kevern, '"I pray that I will not fall over the edge": what is left of faith after dementia?', *Practical Theology* 4 (2011), pp. 283–94, 286.

12 J. Swinton, *Dementia: Living in the Memories of God*, London: SCM Press, 2012, p. 21.

GOD IN FRAGMENTS

thirties and forties with early-onset dementia who, faced with
a poor prognosis, diminishing abilities and young children, are
taking pictures and videos and having experiences that will,
they hope, allow their children to remember them when they
are gone. Many non-clinical studies are now collecting the
thoughts of people with dementia in context.[13] Russell sees this
principle as a way of re-thinking our attitudes on the basis
of the way people with dementia express themselves, arguing
that our relationships with other people are in some ways like
our relationship with God.[14] For some people, such a coherent
expression of their feelings may not be possible. John Swinton's
acquaintance 'Stephen', with Down's syndrome, 'has limited
verbal skills and different cognitive functioning, so his experience of the world is not limited by the context of words'. Yet
our inclination is ever to place 'reason, intellect, and rationality
above emotion, intuition, and experience'.[15] Are we letting our
own experiences of worship, and our understanding of what
we are doing, get in the way of understanding and accepting
the way that others do the same thing? Is this perhaps endemic
in the Church in any case? Our prejudices are not limited to
the experiences of people who are not 'neurotypical'. But the
stories of each person with dementia are particular to their circumstances, and their experiences and abilities in the context of
worship may vary dramatically day by day or over the course
of years. Telling these stories is an important way of emphasiz-
ing the unique experiences of each person of God. They help us
on our own journey of discipleship because they emphasize for
us the diversity and fragility of the Body of Christ. In the next
section, we re-evaluate the merits and benefits of worshipping
alongside the whole Church of God – cohesive and welcoming
– and consider the goals and expectations of our worship more
generally.

13 See Kevern, Russell, Swinton, Kennedy, Higgins.
14 Russell, 'Listening to dementia', pp. 17–18.
15 Swinton, *Dementia*, p. 3.

44

Re-imagining participation

Traditional impressions of liturgical participation and engagement need to be re-framed for people with dementia, who may behave or react unconventionally, but help us to shape our understanding of what it means to live authentically for the worship of God.

With Alison Phinney, we ask, 'How do people, even in the midst of the profound breakdown of dementia, go about living a life of meaning and worth?'[16] Some might ask, can one even 'be a Christian' when one changes as a consequence of dementia? Does one still satisfy the same 'demanding criteria for church membership', and is that person still 'in possession of the same salvation?'[17] God *qua* God is often thought of as analogous to

> a conscious mind; and the action of God on believers has frequently been understood . . . in terms of their conscious perception of God, intellectual assent to divine authority and response through intentional activity. Since the capacities to perceive, assent, and respond intentionally appear to be progressively lost as a person's dementia progresses, questions inevitably arise about their status as a Christian and the goodness of the God they serve.[18]

Confessing Jesus as Lord, the basic tenet of the faith, requires 'a certain level of subjectivity, awareness, and cognitive competence'.[19] Yet this assumption sits uncomfortably, since people with dementia, at least at the early and advancing stages, are able to articulate their understanding of spiritual practices: in the words of Gladys, interviewed by Higgins, in prayer 'I'm talking to the Lord and he's talking back to me . . . The Lord has picked up a passage [of the Bible] and spoken to me.'[20]

---

16 Phinney, 'Horizons of meaning', p. 254.

17 Kevern, 'Grace of foolishness', p. 207.

18 Kevern, 'I pray that . . .', p. 284.

19 Swinton, *Dementia*, p. 161.

20 P. Higgins, '"It's a consolation": the role of Christian religion for people with dementia who are living in care homes', *Journal of Religion, Spirituality and Aging* 26 (2014), pp. 320–39.

For others, familiar childhood prayers said over a lifetime are frequently repeated and spoken of as a source of comfort.[21] In another study the spouse of a man with dementia said that reading Scripture to him was a comfort when he woke up with night terrors and confusion.[22] Some people with dementia who have cared for others still have the desire to help people, or to minister to them, sometimes but not always in the way they had done earlier in their lives.[23] Surely this illustrates and illuminates their continuing vocation as a Christian.

Sometimes the use of familiar prayers and phrases is dismissed on the grounds that people with dementia 'don't know what they are saying', that the phrases are, using the terminology of J. L. Austin, 'phatic' utterances like 'how do you do?' and 'I hope you slept well'.[24] Yet such remarks would be less well tolerated if applied to children, who, it might be argued, also have little sense of what they are saying. But is it always the case that 'neurotypical' adults always mean what they say in the liturgy ('Peace be with you') or that we always engage prayerfully and powerfully with the Lord's Prayer?

Malcolm Goldsmith reminds us that we also develop sometimes very complicated and entertaining bedtime rituals with our dogs, as well as unspoken rules and conventions among families, especially at times like Christmas: presents before or after lunch?[25] The value and centrality of ritual in our lives, while often scorned as something pertaining to a particular constituency (within the Church or otherwise), ought to be

21 Higgins, 'It's a consolation', pp. 331–2.
22 Phinney, 'Horizons of meaning', p. 263.
23 Higgins, 'It's a consolation', p. 327.
24 For Austin's theory of the 'phatic' or habitual performative utterance, see J. L. Austin, *How to Do Things with Words*, Oxford: Clarendon Press, 1962, pp. 95–6. The term 'phatic communion' was used first by Bronislaw Malinowski, in 'The problem of meaning in primitive languages', in C. K. Ogden and I. A. Richards (eds), *The Meaning of Meaning: A Study of the Influence of Languages upon Thought and the Science of Symbolism*, London: Kegan Paul, 1923.
25 M. Goldsmith, 'When words are no longer necessary: the gift of ritual', *Journal of Religious Gerontology* 12 (2002), pp. 139–50, 140, 145.

something that we accept and embrace. We are surrounded by rituals of sorts in all our activities, many of which are in theory optional and not necessary for the success of the activity – from laying the dinner table in a particular way, to getting down on one knee (or expecting someone to get down on one knee) to propose marriage. Others help us to remember to do something that is good, like brushing one's teeth. Like all of us, people with dementia have lived lives full of these rituals and, entirely apart from the displacement that comes naturally with entering an institution, it is probably very disconcerting to be divested of the particular daily conventions that don't work in that environment. For Goldsmith, dementia itself is 'a violation of the ceremonial rules of everyday life', so there is value in retaining such rituals as may be expedient.[26] Patricia Suggs points out the possibility of creating new rituals that commemorate significant events in the context of care.[27] Among the rituals she proposes are:

- a ceremony to bless and empower the work of caregivers and care workers;
- a Memory Bridge building a connection between a person with dementia, their family and caregivers, and the care facility that they are now entering;
- a 'ritual of passage', or crossing the threshold, for those moving to another level of care; small rituals for someone who has been told bad news, for mealtimes, for the death of a resident or staff member, or for the loss of a physical function.

It is the sometimes very different ways in which people with dementia engage with ritual that can be unsettling both to them and to those who worship with them. This is true whether in a 'high church' environment or in charismatic services: both have their own rituals and common expectations of the worshipper.

---

26 Goldsmith, 'When words', p. 144.
27 P. K. Suggs and D. L. Suggs, 'The understanding and creation of rituals: enhancing the life of older adults', *Journal of Religious Gerontology* 15 (2003), pp. 17–24, 22.

While we may tend to be most critical of worship that requires reading and following along on a service sheet, the conventions of freer forms of worship are equally pervasive. In the worship environment, we typically prioritize agency and the ability to express oneself as intrinsic to personhood, as well as a precondition for the work of the gospel that every Christian is compelled to perform. Similarly, the efficacy of the worship of the Christian in church has so often been judged on the basis of worshippers' active participation in the words and other aspects of services. This view has dominated since the beginning of the so-called 'Liturgical Movement' of the later nineteenth century. After the promulgation of the documents on the liturgy issued by the Second Vatican Council in the 1960s, joining in with the words, songs and prayers came to be seen by many, across a wide range of churches, as the aspired-for goal that would serve congregations spiritually and make their numbers rise. This understanding of vocalization as participation does not sit well with the experiences of many people with dementia. It is here argued that on a more general level, and especially in the case of people with dementia, we need to give greater credence in this regard to prayerful engagement, whether audible or not, and whether in synchrony with others or not, with the work of the Body of Christ, in ways that may not always cohere with this kind of participation. In the words of Lyndal Vaught, worship ought to be 'a dialogue of God's revelation and the worshipper's response',[28] but the response may take many forms – just as it does for 'neurotypical' people. Indeed, do we presume to understand the mystery of the liturgy at which we are present? Our own presumptions about how successfully we ourselves participate in and benefit from the liturgy could stand being evaluated from time to time, and our own assumptions about how our own practices sit well with others might well be reconsidered.

Australian biochemist and former government adviser Christine Bryden developed symptoms of dementia at the age of 46 and has since become a well-known author and speaker

---

28 L. Vaught, 'Worship models and music in spiritual formation', *Journal of Religion, Spirituality and Aging* 22 (2009), pp. 104–19, 107.

on the subject, her latest book being *Will I Still Be Me?*[29] She writes elsewhere, 'I may not be able to take an active part in worship, but I can receive the gifts of love and grace. This is the good news of the Gospel for those of us living with dementia: we are equal before God in receiving divine love and grace.'[30] We overlook ways of relating because we prioritize 'rational behaviour' and apparent cognition as integral to the life of a Christian.

The person with dementia is present, together with the rest of us, in a worship environment full of complex multisensory expectations. It is striking that the success of our active participation, and by extension the success of our worship, is often measured by our satisfying the norms for vocalization, movement and posture. As mentioned above, the Roman Catholic Constitution on the Sacred Liturgy, *Sacrosanctum Concilium* (1963), has often been held responsible for this unhelpful attitude, but this is a misunderstanding and an unhelpful explanation of the Council's position. *Sacrosanctum Concilium* ordered that the laity should be exhorted to attend services 'knowingly, actively, and fruitfully', with their minds focused on the rites being celebrated. For all, 'the very nature of the Liturgy' demands 'full, conscious, and active participation', for this is 'the primary and indispensable source from which the faithful are to derive the true Christian spirit'. At other times, those present were to observe a 'reverent silence'. In the decades that followed, 'full and active participation' became a mantra that justified liturgical reform in every possible direction, as long as it appeared to encourage the understanding or a visibly or audibly active role for those in the congregation. The renewed liturgical structures of all churches have become testing-grounds for patterns of words and actions that change regularly and that are governed by rules beyond the ken of typical worshippers. The Church of England's contemporary

---

29 C. Bryden, *Will I Still Be Me? Finding a Continuing Sense of Self in the Lived Experience of Dementia*, London: Jessica Kingsley Publishers, 2018.

30 C. Bryden, 'Letter to the Church', *Journal of Disability and Religion* 22 (2018), pp. 96–106, 105.

liturgical structures have been part of this impulse towards variability: today's *Common Worship* rites, while they might in many places be broadly indistinguishable from Roman Catholic, Lutheran or Methodist equivalents, also follow the ecumenical consensus in embracing the foundational principle of 'freedom within a framework', allowing within the basic liturgical structures a plethora of textual and ritual options.

People with dementia may find it difficult at times to adhere to the norms of the congregation, even if the form of service is familiar, and their frustration may be greatly amplified if, within familiar structures, the ways in which they are expected to participate are changed, season by season or even week by week (or day by day). While it is attractive for our liturgy to reflect the richness of Christian tradition and creativity, we should be careful that our expectations of active participation by people who cannot readily read and appreciate the contents of a service booklet are appropriate to the context. In fact, if we would like our congregations in general to engage productively with the words of our worship, we might do well to restrict the range of options that we use, so that all might be able to pray by heart, from the heart.

Subsequent chapters deal in greater detail with the challenges and opportunities of crafting liturgical material that is 'dementia-friendly', or for worship in homes or care homes or other special contexts. However, many of the positive features of worship that is dementia-friendly agree with the general principles of worship 'in spirit and in truth' – that is, worship that builds up the Body of Christ. In such worship, a person with dementia may recognize or be able to join in with prayers, actions and sentiments through their presence and awareness, even if they cannot communicate in the accepted way, and even if the gathered community is not itself present.

It is often suggested that stimuli such as music, dance and art are important ways of engaging people with cognitive difficulties, and particularly with dementia where they may be able to elicit memories and bring people into 'the moment'. In the 1950s Anton Boisen, an American healthcare chaplain, wrote, 'The purpose of worship is to help us face our actual problems and difficulties in the light of Christian faith and thus to find insight and courage to deal with them effectively.' Boisen was involved in the early development of the 'clinical pastoral movement' and also produced his own hymnal, *Hymns of Hope and Courage*, designed for use by the mentally ill. He believed that, at heart, it should not matter whether hymns were being chosen for 'mental patients or [for] persons who are presumably normal'. In general, the words rather than the tunes were significant (the tunes being 'therapeutically neutral').[31] In the study inspired by Boisen's work, Eldred and colleagues observed that subjects, primarily older women, 'reported that certain hymns can raise their spirits and that this was usually due to the combination of the words and the tunes of the hymns, experienced by singing them'.[32] In reference to the frequent suggestion that (so to speak) traditional hymns and words should be sung, they recognized the possible difficulties arising from the lack of uniformity in worship or styles of preferred music, and a diminished sense of history, although (in the words of a 90-year-old) 'new hymns will be the memories of today's young'.[33] Another study argues that not only do people with dementia respond better (how so?) to familiar music, the use of 'music' rather than 'music therapy' needs to be distinguished.

How should we understand our own role in planning and participating in worship? For many worshippers with dementia, the answers are clear, nowhere more so than in a 'Letter to the Church' appropriating the form of a Pauline epistle, written by Christine Bryden.[34] She writes, 'I want to encourage my friends in the church to look to our continuing sense of being an embodied self in relationship with God and within the community, and help us to search for meaning in the present

---

31 J. B. Eldred et al., 'Your heart can dance to them even if your feet can't', *Practical Theology* 7 (2014), pp. 153–79, 160, 161, 164.

32 Eldred et al., 'Your heart can dance', p. 166.

33 Eldred et al., 'Your heart can dance', pp. 170, 173.

34 C. Bryden, *Who Will I Be When I Die?*, London: Jessica Kingsley Publishers, 2012; and C. Bryden, *Dancing with Dementia*, London: Jessica Kingsley Publishers, 2005.

moment.'[35] Bryden reminds the Church that Jesus came for all, 'not just for those with cognitive capacity'. There is no relationship of direct proportion between cognition and the need for Jesus, just as there is no 'normal' set of human circumstances against which all others are compared. She notes that Jesus taught us to pray 'Our Father . . . give us this day our daily bread' and so on.[36] In Bryden's view of the Church, 'there is no need for cognition, for this is a spiritual communion':[37] all are called to relate to each of the other members of the body in this spiritual communion, even those with dementia and even those whose behaviour and capacities are changing. She writes, 'I seek the simple gift of the community's presence, to watch, wait, and pray, as Jesus asked of the disciples in the Garden of Gethsemane', a state where silence, as well as gesture and touch, are important means of communion.[38]

In the Garden of Gethsemane Jesus asks his disciples to stay and watch with him. The disciples, perhaps because they are weary and fearful, fall asleep, while Jesus prays to his Father to let the cup pass from him. There is much in Christine Bryden's request: that we stay close to those among us who ask for our prayers and company, even in times of great stress and sorrow, and that in being attentive to their needs we do not 'fall asleep'. The disciples did not manage it for Jesus. The spirit is willing, but the flesh is weak.

Learning from people with dementia

What do we all learn about God and the Church when we worship alongside people with dementia? In worship, in the gathered Body of Christ, we see and join with all the parts of that body (in weakness is God's strength), and are formed ourselves. It is in this Body of Christ, expressing its response to God's work in us, that we see the full and authentic contribution

35 Bryden, 'Letter', p. 96.
36 Bryden, 'Letter', p. 98.
37 Bryden, 'Letter', p. 99.
38 Bryden, 'Letter', p. 103.

of the person living with dementia. Each one of us is formed and shaped by our collective participation. God is often to be seen in weakness.

It is axiomatic that when the Christian community comes together to pray, the diversity of the many members of the Body of Christ may be seen. Each has their own particular abilities and strengths, and each has their role to play in that community. The worship offered by that commmunity, too, has an essential role in shaping and structuring its life.[39] In the Body of Christ, and especially in the sacraments, the people of God are united to Christ and to one another. As Paul writes, 'For in the one Spirit we were all baptized into one body' (1 Corinthians 12.13). Partaking of Christ's body in its sacramental presence is in particular a way of being taken up into this communion: 'We who are many are one body, for we all partake of the one bread' (1 Corinthians 10.17). Equally, the community is only as strong as each one of its members, and all are affected by the experiences of a single member. 'If one member suffers, all suffer together with it' (1 Corinthians 12.26).

It is just as axiomatic that we should love and serve the Lord in our interactions and attitudes when we worship: as the Liturgical Commission has written, 'We must not let the familiar words of the Dismissal mislead us into thinking that, while we are still at worship, our active service to the world and to one another has not yet begun.'[40] As we walk alongside those with dementia Matthew 25.40 comes to mind: 'Just as you did it to one of the least of these . . . you did it to me.'

How do we change our habits of worship to walk alongside people with dementia, and what might we gain in doing so? The liturgical scholar Romano Guardini argued at the time of the Second Vatican Council that liturgical renewal was not just about changing the words or the ways that churches were built. Rather, the most important aspect of renewal was helping people to re-learn how to do some of the simplest actions.

---

39 *Transforming Worship: Living the New Creation. A Report by the Liturgical Commission* (GS 1651), Archbishops' Council, 2007, 2.9.

40 *Transforming Worship*, 2.3.

In a similar way but for very different reasons, John Swinton writes, 'Each human encounter is an occasion for worship: an opportunity to place our bodies in particular ways before God and for the other . . . Worship provides a space within which the Body of Christ can take shape and form as it seeks to respond faithfully to the calling of Jesus.'[41] What insights might we gain by opening ourselves up in this way?

Several writers have recognized the resonance of the imagery of sheep and shepherd for many people with dementia, who may feel 'lost' or in need of guidance or leading: Psalm 23, but also the ninety-nine sheep and the one, as well as Christ as the Good Shepherd. The Spirit who dwells in God's temple (1 Corinthians 3.16) is also foundational. Perpetual membership of the flock, and the continued exercise of that right, is of great importance. Christians are baptized into one Body, and (for Swinton) lose ownership of their own bodies as they become one in Christ. The flock is led by the shepherd. Swinton writes, 'It is not that our individual bodies cease to matter. They actually become more important as they find their true *telos*.'[42] In interviews, people of faith with dementia articulate that they know that 'what is happening now is *only temporary and will pale in significance in comparison when they reach their heavenly home*'.[43]

Swinton writes, 'Worship is something that we do with our bodies. Worship occurs when we position our bodies in particular ways before the Creator and allow the Spirit to open our heart to the transforming rhythm of God's intentions.' More importantly, worship ought to shape and build up the community as the Body of Christ, dependent on its constituent members whatever their condition. 'Bodies matter to Christians. At the heart of our faith is the broken body of Jesus. It is as we look upon the damaged body of Jesus on the cross that we come to realize that God is and remains embodied.'[44]

---

41 Swinton, *Dementia*, p. 236.
42 Swinton, *Dementia*, p. 231.
43 Higgins, 'It's a consolation', p. 333 (emphasis added).
44 Swinton, *Dementia*, pp. 228–9.

If I must boast, I will boast of the things that show my weakness. (2 Corinthians 11.30)

For he was crucified in weakness, but lives by the power of God. For we are weak in him, but in dealing with you we will live with him by the power of God. (2 Corinthians 13.4)

Paul says 'I boast' 19 times in chapters 10 to 13 of 2 Corinthians: here he boasts of his own weakness, incapacity and failure which provide the opportunity for God's grace in Christ to be manifest. In sum, he boasts that human weakness is God's strength:

So, I will boast all the more gladly of my weaknesses, so that the power of Christ may dwell in me. Therefore I am content with weaknesses, insults, hardships, persecutions, and calamities for the sake of Christ; for whenever I am weak, then I am strong. (2 Corinthians 12.9b–10)

The 'dependency, neediness, and interconnectedness' that remind us of the Trinity are also characteristics of people with dementia, people who are part of the whole, good creation of God. In so seeing and participating in worship with people with dementia, we are being formed and shaped, and they are being upheld and remain welcome in their community.

What might we learn from people with dementia? How do they enrich the lives of their congregations? At least one commentator (Peter Kevern) references the idea of the 'holy fool', a term that is perhaps unfortunate but a concept that may be quite productive. In the tradition of devotional literature, the holy fool was someone who behaved eccentrically but who was, in fact, divinely inspired. Kevern refers to Leontius' *Life of Symeon the Holy Fool* as an example of the concept: someone who seems to behave irrationally, but whose behaviour is caused by a higher spiritual motivation. 'Symeon appears bad, but is good; respectable Christian society appears good, but is blind and ignorant.'[45] The holy fool often appears at the margins of society. In the spirit of Christian *koinonia*

---

45 Kevern, 'Grace of foolishness', pp. 211–13.

(joint-participation, sharing), we should resist making 'the dementia service', or accommodations to make our worship 'dementia-friendly', part of the margins of our community, even if people do things that might make us feel uncomfortable or alarmed, behaviour that seems 'superficially very unholy'.[46] Swinton reports the horrified reaction of one minister administering communion, in the presence of a woman with Down's syndrome: 'Don't let that woman take the sacrament! She will defile it.'[47] Yet a variety of accounts show that if it formed an important part of their life before the onset of dementia, taking communion remains a significant part of a person's spiritual life. Reflecting that no one understands any more than Stephen what the Eucharist might really be, Swinton writes, 'One of Stephen's main problems is not his cognitive deficits or "behavioural difficulties", but rather the inability of those around him to understand his life experiences and to treat him with the respect and dignity that his status as a human being demands.'[48]

Paul expresses something essential about the diversity of the Church in chapter 12 of 1 Corinthians.[49] He is calling on the Church to understand the interdependence, and unity, of the members of Christ in a single body. First, the community of the Church is itself linked to this body with many diverse components, each with its own function (verse 12). Second, the members of the body are diverse, with diverse functions, but are mutually supportive and interdependent: 'If the whole body were an eye, where would the hearing be?' (verse 17). In fact, the weaker members of the body are 'indispensable' and need special care that the stronger parts do not need. And yet all are dependent on one another: 'The eye cannot say to the hand, "I have no need of you", nor again the head to the feet, "I have no need of you"' (verse 21). All parts of the Church have the right and need to be upheld and supported for the better of the whole.

---

46 Kevern, 'Grace of foolishness', p. 209.
47 Swinton, *Dementia*, p. 234.
48 Swinton, *Dementia*, pp. 9, 31.
49 And cf. Romans 12, Ephesians 4, Colossians 2.

The Christian approach to sickness cannot help but exist in the shadow of the healing miracles of Jesus, in which great suffering is ameliorated for those who believe: indeed, Jesus says that 'all things can be done for the one who believes'. This assertion, from chapter 9 of Mark's Gospel, happens during Jesus' intervention in the healing of the boy with an unclean spirit. The disciples have not been able to cast out the spirit, and in frustration the boy's father reports this fact to Jesus. In a beautiful and memorable exclamation, he cries, 'I believe; help my unbelief!' The disciples, too, are perplexed, and enquire why they had not been able to heal the boy. Jesus replies, 'This kind can come out only through prayer.' Imagine the reaction of the disciples: have they not been trying through prayer? When we pray for people with dementia, and their condition does not improve markedly, do we not identify with these disciples?

It might be thought insensitive to compare the condition of this boy (described in Matthew 17 as epilepsy) with the suffering of a person with dementia, but there are some interesting parallels. The boy has a 'mute spirit', *pneuma alalon*, which prohibits him from speaking. One can easily understand the frustration of the disciples and of the boy's father at fruitless attempts at making the situation better. We may be frustrated, too, that despite our prayers and best efforts at accommodation, a person with dementia is still confused, excluded, and spiritually troubled in worship. What more could we do?

The disciples might have been confused further by the fact that despite Jesus' assertion that the boy could only be delivered through prayer, no prayer seems to have happened. Instead, the story points to the confession of faithlessness of the boy's father. Joel Marcus writes, 'The gap between the two levels of the Markan narrative, then, is bridged both by seeing the church's prayer as an expression of faith and by seeing the father's supplication before Jesus, which is faithful in its very confession of faithlessness, as a kind of prayer.'[50] Faith for Mark is not just the faith of the person who wills that some-

---

50 J. Marcus, *Mark 8—16: A New Translation with Introduction and Commentary*, New Haven, CT: Yale University Press, 2009, p. 665.

thing should be done, but the 'total human context in which a potential miracle might take place ... The man's famous reply [I believe – help my unbelief!] shows that faith is both a human response and a gift from outside ... Faith for Mark is the absolute trust and dependence on God which can be and is reflected precisely in the activity of prayer.'[51]

As is the case with some people with dementia, the boy was like a corpse. But Jesus took him, lifted him up, and he was able to stand. Jesus will lift up all the faithful by his being lifted high on the cross.

Reflecting on the act of worshipping alongside someone with complex needs, John Swinton writes, 'When we encounter [him] we are faced with a deep revelation of the nature of God as we are reminded of the dependency, neediness, and interconnectedness that is a mark of the very being of the Trinitarian God. Human beings made in God's image are interdependent creatures: dependent on God and dependent on one another.'[52]

What can members of the congregation do? Looking eagerly forward to the presence of Jesus in their midst, they can, if practical, attend worship in the care home or hospital, or help materially with services in church where people with dementia are likely to be present. It is in the context of a medical or care facility, in particular, that there is no Jew or Greek, male or female.[53] Here, particularly where the facility is not a religious foundation, there may be a misconception that spiritual care has been 'done' if there is a church service, and that if there is no religious foundation, no spiritual need should ever be addressed. It is seen as the responsibility of chaplains and church contacts, but without meaningful contact with an ecclesial community, even with its minister alone, an element is lost.[54] Bryden reminds the Church that, in the words of Jesus,

---

51 J. Barton and J. Muddiman (eds), *Oxford Bible Commentary*, Oxford: Oxford University Press, 2007; Mark 9.14–29.

52 J. Swinton, 'Building a Church for strangers', *Journal of Religion, Disability & Health* 4 (2001), pp. 25–63, 45.

53 Swinton, *Dementia*, p. 5.

54 M. A. Goodall, 'The evaluation of spiritual care in a dementia care setting', *Dementia* 8 (2009), pp. 167–83, 169.

who spoke with children and outcasts, 'just as you did it to one of the least of these who are members of my family, you did it to me' (Matthew 25.40). When this radical work is done, Jesus is truly in the midst of the faithful.

In 2 Corinthians Paul writes:

> But we have this treasure in clay jars, so that it may be made clear that this extraordinary power belongs to God and does not come from us. We are afflicted in every way, but not crushed; perplexed, but not driven to despair; persecuted, but not forsaken; struck down, but not destroyed; always carrying in the body the death of Jesus, so that the life of Jesus may also be made visible in our bodies. For while we live, we are always being given up to death for Jesus' sake, so that the life of Jesus may be made visible in our mortal flesh. So death is at work in us, but life in you. (2 Corinthians 4.7–12)

Our own bodies, as well as those with whom we walk, are incomplete, insufficient vessels in which to hold Christ, and their capacity for failure, misfortune and affliction is the means by which that divine Presence is made known. In these insufficiencies God gives Paul, and all of us, the capacity to know his grace and love in Christ so that we may live. When we gather in community, we have the opportunity to see every kind of clay jar, each one fragile and not up to the complete task. In such a way, when we worship alongside people with dementia, we stand as equal – and equally weak – children of God. In the darkness of the garden of Gethsemane, Christ's bloody tears and sweat are visible to us. As Robert Davis, a retired pastor with dementia, has put it, 'I can look beyond the moonlight and see glorious "Sonlight" emanating from the Son of God himself enthroned in that place where all things are changed to become perfect – heaven.'[55]

---

55 Kevern, 'I pray that I will not fall over the edge', p. 288.

4

Creating Dementia-friendly Worship

JULIA BURTON-JONES

This chapter introduces you to innovative approaches that have
been developed in recent years to enable people with dementia to continue to worship. The first part of the chapter gives
a brief overview of ways in which liturgy and service design
might be adapted to accommodate those with different cognitive abilities. This might involve changes to regular worship
but could also include offering special services designed around
the needs of people with dementia, worshipping in a church
building but also in the places people live. Three case studies
are then presented to illustrate creative ways of worshipping
that fully engage people who may struggle with thinking and
remembering.

Aspects of worship that might be challenging

Everyone with dementia is different, so it would be wrong to
generalize here about how a person may experience a church
service. Dementia is a progressive condition and the symptoms
are mild early on; participating in worship may not pose
difficulties for those with a recent diagnosis. As symptoms
become more noticeable, fellow members of the congregation
might pick up that the person is finding it hard to follow the
pattern of a service. Concentration flags somewhat and there is
uncertainty over what to do when. If you examine the average
church service, you will find that it holds plenty of cognitive
challenge. Services tend to be wordy, and you might move from

one book to another at various points. There are unwritten rules about when to sit and when to stand, when to be quiet and when to talk. The message or sermon may require considerable attention and understanding of sometimes abstract ideas.

In later dementia the typical format for worship can be difficult. Here are some common scenarios:

- The service is too long for a person whose concentration is limited.
- The service does not engage the person because it is pitched at a cerebral level that is challenging.
- The service involves the congregation following an unspoken pattern of responses and behaviour that the person struggles to follow and remember.
- The service is largely word-based, when language skills are faltering in dementia; elements that engage the senses and involve movement are limited, whereas it is these aspects that hold the power still to evoke a response.
- Boredom may prompt the person to get up and walk out, causing what friends and family members perceive to be disruption.
- The service requires periods of silence that the person does not understand; they make noises that embarrass friends and relatives accompanying them.
- The service is bewildering for a person who finds it difficult to filter out unwanted noises and they can become distressed through over-stimulation.
- The service draws from recent liturgy and music that the person can neither recall nor learn because of impaired short-term memory; their memory of songs and prayers learned in early life is what remains.
- The person feels anxious in what may seem an unfamiliar environment, and the opportunity for friends and family members to provide reassurance is limited by the context.

Elements to include in accessible worship and principles to consider

The case studies below illustrate how, through incorporating dementia-friendly liturgy, we can enable people to continue to flourish in worship, finding it a source of joy and encouragement. Here are some principles drawn from the case studies that are worth considering, both in adapting regular worship, and in designing services aimed at people with dementia.

Creating an atmosphere conducive to worship – people with dementia may find it difficult to comprehend what is happening at an intellectual level, while their ability to make sense of the relational aspects of a situation remain intact. They will be attuned to the warmth of welcome they receive, and sensitive to attitudes and responses that are belittling. Helping those who come to worship to feel settled and safe is a key goal, so considering seating arrangements and strategies for ensuring no one feels stranded and alone, through named welcomers or 'buddies', is helpful. The physical environment may also be a prompt to worship, with music and visual prompts that give clues and set the tone of what is about to happen.

Drawing from the person's Christian heritage – the process of memory loss in dementia means that the person's more recent memories are lost first; over time experiences that can be most easily recalled are from earlier in their life. Prayers and songs they were familiar with in middle and later life might be forgotten, but Bible passages and choruses learned in Sunday school are still remembered. Including hymns familiar from childhood in services sparks those early memories. Using older versions of Scripture and prayer books may be useful, such as the old version of the Lord's Prayer, which seems to be held in the memory until very late in dementia, bringing a response even from those for whom verbal communication has become very limited.

Using music effectively – research shows that music has the capacity to reach people with dementia when other means of engaging with them have little effect.[1] This is because it draws upon particular areas of the brain that are less damaged in dementia. Incorporating music in worship is important. Singing has many benefits for people with dementia.[2]

Participatory approaches – sitting passively through services has limited value for people who are struggling to concentrate and follow what is being said. The case studies below all illustrate the need to engage people with dementia actively in exploring Christian themes. Through group discussion, singing together and craft work, for example, participants with dementia can engage in the act of worship and derive meaning and encouragement.

Reminiscence – drawing on memories of early life in the style of reminiscence therapy is also helpful in introducing a Christian theme. This can be done through looking at objects and pictures related to the theme. It allows the person to feel valued in their perspectives and experiences, and to add to the group's understanding of the topic. It opens the heart and spirit to how the Bible sheds light on issues of everyday life.

Simplicity, familiarity and pacing – following a regular pattern of worship allows people with dementia to become familiar with the form you are using. Use simple liturgies, expressing the truths of our faith in ways that can easily be grasped. Avoid abstract ideas and obscure language. Make good use of silence, to allow someone whose brain is working more slowly to process what is happening; speak at a measured pace, not rushing between activities but explaining clearly what comes next.

---

1 S. M. Bamford and S. Bowell, 'What would life be – without a song or a dance, what are we?', *A Report from the Commission on Dementia and Music*, International Longevity Centre, 2018.

2 T. Vella-Burrows, *Singing and People with Dementia*, Sidney De Haan Research Centre for Arts and Health, 2012.

Working with all the senses – we know that people with dementia increasingly experience the world around them through their senses. Engaging the senses is a good way to make a connection and spark interest and understanding.

Creativity – in working with people with dementia, worship leaders have discovered that creative, arts-based approaches prove effective. This might include a craft activity around the theme of the session (as in Messy Vintage, described below), or using movement and dance.[3]

Story-telling – bibliotherapy, where stories and poems are read or created together, has been found to engage and provide a calming context for people living with dementia. Godly Play (as used in Stories for the Soul – Case Study 2) is a good example of this.

Giving as well as receiving – people with dementia have the ability and desire to continue to minister to those around them, so opportunities for them to be a blessing within their Christian family are enriching for us all. This may be continuing in roles they previously fulfilled, with some support and prompting, or new areas of ministry. Ministers report that a direct line to the heart of God is still very much in evidence when people in late dementia pray aloud, finding a fluency that is not generally seen in their day-to-day conversations.

---

3 All Party Parliamentary Group on Arts, Health and Wellbeing, *Creative Health: The Arts for Health and Wellbeing*, 2017.

CASE STUDY 1: ST MATTHEW'S CHURCH IN WIGMORE, GILLINGHAM

(Written with the Revd Brian Senior, Sue Jelfs and Jean Penney)

St Matthew's is one of four churches in the benefice of South Gillingham in Medway. It sits in a residential neighbourhood and has a high proportion of older members, several of whom are living with dementia.

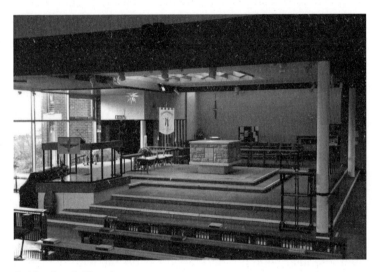

St Matthew's Church

It was this experience of dementia among congregation members that awakened the church to the need to adjust their usual patterns of worship. Being alongside several people through their dementia has shaped and informed responses, so when the diocese ran a project on 'dementia-friendly churches' in 2014, South Gillingham was one of the parishes most actively involved, hosting several 'Dementia Friends' sessions for the deanery that were attended by many members of the congregation.

Three key people in the parish played a vital role in establishing a monthly dementia-friendly church service. Jean Penney, church warden and recently retired social worker, saw how Alzheimer's affected her own father, and her mum as his carer. Lay reader Sue Jelfs was working as pastoral care co-ordinator in a local Christian care home for people with dementia, after a career in nursing. Rector Brian Senior reflected on the experience of his mum's dementia, and being the father of a young man with Down's syndrome, in understanding the perspectives of congregation members facing cognitive challenges. Between them Jean, Sue and Brian identified both a need and an opportunity to respond positively.

Consulting people with dementia and their carers after hosting Dementia Friends sessions, St Matthew's picked up a need for more information about the help available locally for people with dementia and their families. With the support of local health and care organizations they planned an information event for April 2016. Many local providers of services displayed information in the hall, giving advice and support, while in the church itself speakers included a local person with young-onset dementia, Lorraine Brown, and a panel of carers organized by the charity Carers First. Refreshments were provided through the day and over 150 people attended. Plans to hold a regular church service aimed at people with dementia were shared at the event, and the first monthly service was scheduled for September 2016.

Dementia-friendly services at St Matthew's are now held on the fourth Wednesday of each month at 2.30 p.m. They have been well attended since the beginning, with an average of 35 worshippers. Several are longstanding members of the church, but many come from other parishes, including some who travel quite a distance. From the outset residents from a Christian dementia care home in nearby Strood have been brought to the service by minibus. Residents from a care home alongside the church also come regularly.

Built in 1965, St Matthew's has a relatively modern building which means it has good access for people with limited mobility. The services are held in the café area of the church which is in the transept alongside the main sanctuary. The team feel it is important to have the service in church, as this helps orientate people living with dementia to the fact that they are taking part in worship. Round tables are laid with colourful cloths and worshippers sit café-style around the tables. An altar is set up with white table linen, a cross and a candle, as a focus and a visual prompt.

Hymns are chosen that are well known by people with dementia, whose long-term memories are more secure than memories of songs they sang in church in later years. Usually three hymns are sung during the service, and the keyboard accompaniment is provided by the former church organist who himself is a person with dementia; having recently relinquished playing in the main Sunday services, he appreciates leading the worship at the Wednesday services.

Each service is based around a theme. These themes were initially selected from the book *Living Liturgies*, by Caroline George (published by the Bible Reading Fellowship in 2015). Everyday objects, such as keys and curtains, are used to spark reflection on biblical stories and truths. This makes the themes relatable and tangible for people with dementia. After an opening hymn, the theme is introduced at the beginning of the service with the aid of pictures and objects placed on the altar. The session on keys, for instance, involved the group looking at many different keys, including keys to the church building. There will be some discussion about the objects used to illustrate the theme where the group can share their memories and ideas. A Bible reading related to the theme follows, and then a short talk led by Brian, Sue or the curate Christine, where the congregation again participate.

After the talk everyone is encouraged to share topics for which they would appreciate prayer. A simple response is used in gathering up these requests ('Lord, in your mercy: hear our prayer'). Prayers finish with the traditional version of the Lord's Prayer. There is a closing hymn and worship finishes with a simple blessing. The service has lasted no more than 30 minutes and is followed by another half-hour of tea, cake and conversation. Faithful volunteers from St Matthew's take responsibility for supplying appetizing cakes each month, which is doubtless part of the draw for those who attend.

Now that a routine has been established and roles shared between volunteers, the service is not felt to be burdensome or a drain on church resources. Jean reflects that the most time-consuming task is setting up the tables and chairs and clearing them afterwards. The parish have a clear strategy for publicizing the service. They distribute posters and postcard-size cards with dates of the year's services in many local venues. The service is also publicized to members of Medway Dementia Action Alliance, so that health and social care professionals now refer people they support with dementia who have expressed a desire to be linked with a church.

Coming to the Wednesday service has encouraged some to come back to church on Sundays. The timing of the main Sunday service has been altered from 9.30 to 10.00 a.m. to allow people who struggle with an early start to attend. Carers have expressed how the regular opportunity to meet with other people in their situation has helped relieve the sense of isolation that can go hand in hand with caring for a person with dementia. For carers it can be stressful bringing the person with dementia to Sunday worship, but the Wednesday service is a context where they can be completely relaxed; they know that unusual behaviours will be accepted and that no one will mind.

Jean reflects that over the years, attitudes in the congregation have changed in a positive direction. She can remember occasions when a person with dementia talking during a quiet part of the service, or singing the wrong notes in hymns, was met with disapproval. The congregation grew in understanding through being alongside members as their dementia progressed, so that expressions of disapproval at perceived inappropriate behaviour would now be unthinkable. Church members were so used to the discordant singing of one person with dementia they noticed when he was not there and missed him! It took time to help the congregation accept that people with dementia could continue to play an active part in worship, and that occasional mistakes were not the end of the world, but now the church feels a much more inclusive community and is richer for this.

Asked to list essential elements in offering a service for people with dementia, the team identified:

- An informal, accepting ethos that is not judgemental of unusual behaviour.
- Tapping into long-term memories of life and faith.
- Choosing relatable themes that have a clear link to Christian truths.
- Offering tea and cake!
- Using humour to create connections and break down barriers.
- Using simple ideas (as you might do in a school assembly), but showing respect for the age and experience of the congregation in style of delivery, and never being patronizing.
- Facilitating active contributions of people with dementia as long as possible.

CASE STUDY 2: STORIES FOR THE SOUL – GODLY PLAY FOR ELDERS
(Written by Kathryn Lord and the Revd Dr Jeremy Clines)

Godly Play – which when used with older people may be usefully retitled 'Stories for the Soul' – offers an alternative and innovative liturgy for people of all ages and needs. (Godly Play has already been mentioned in Chapter 2.) An international three-year project (2016–18) on 'Godly Play with Elders' is discovering the many benefits that it brings – including being especially significant for the wellbeing of people who are living with dementia.

Godly Play is a creative and imaginative approach to Christian nurture and spiritual life developed by the theologian and educationalist Jerome Berryman.[4] The Godly Play method is centred on the pioneering educational work of Italy's female physician and educator Maria Montessori who, in the 1930s, worked in an asylum and in slums with children who were considered by most people at the time to be unteachable. She discovered that these children could be reached by engaging their hands and their senses. She found and followed the strengths, interests and passions of the children and created the right environment for them to flourish. Berryman developed the Godly Play method for children, basing it upon Montessorian person-centred values, but the method brings spiritual nurture for all participants of any age.

A familiar liturgical pattern is used as the process for every Godly Play session:

1 *Gathering*: each person is individually welcomed as they join a physical circle, overseen by a storyteller and doorperson.
2 *Preparation*: the community is built both by the storyteller and doorperson and also peer-to-peer, and people are helped to get ready with a song or prayer.
3 *Word*: the storyteller presents a story – often biblical or about the Christian tradition – using sensorial and kinaesthetic materials.
4 *Wondering*: the story is reflected upon as a group.

---

4 J. W. Berryman, *Teaching Godly Play: How to Mentor the Spiritual Development of Children*, New York: Morehouse Education Resources, 2009.

5 *Response Time*: the participants are invited to a time to express meaning – for example, by painting, reading, writing, playing, talking and praying.
6 *Feast*: food and drink are enjoyed together – with prayers and perhaps songs – before a final blessing.

The 'wondering' and 'responding' to the Bible's sacred stories is, in fact, a contemporary expression of the ancient spiritual practice of *lectio divina*. Instead of meditating abstractly on Christian Scriptures, there is opportunity for play (in the true sense of the word) in a creative and kinaesthetic way. The creative process of Godly Play is a means for people to explore – verbally and non-verbally – questions that include existential meaning; spiritual identity; how to belong to the Church; life-skills; acquisition of language that helps relate the religious and secular aspects of a person's identity.

The method affirms and honours elements in the Christian tradition that have been less evident in recent centuries: non-verbal communication, quietness, receptivity, awe and wonder. The practice models kindness and mutuality by how it organizes space, materials, and the community of people, and seeks to embody the biblical ethic of how the people of God are to live together.

Godly Play as a participatory liturgy for people living with dementia

A Sheffield 'Godly Play UK' project – which is looking at how the method can bring spiritual wellbeing to people in all areas of the Church's ministry – chose one of its priorities as ministry with older people in care settings, including those living with dementia. There was encouraging anecdotal evidence from others in the UK who were beginning to try out this method, as well as evidence from Lois Howard's ministry over 11 years in the USA.[5] With funding from local and national providers, the Sheffield project is being tried and tested week by week in a variety of care settings in Sheffield and internationally: nursing homes, residential independent living, mental health chaplaincy, dementia cafés and church-based groups. The majority of these are care settings for people living with dementia.

The method creates an environment that belongs to the circle of participants and the spiritual accompaniers are guests in the care setting who wish to enable participation and hospitality from the position of guest. It is apparent that many needs are being addressed within a liturgy that enables mutuality and empowerment: the valuing of individuals and the building of community; reminiscence; mental and spiritual health support; maintaining self and purpose.

Practice narratives

What follows are some practice narratives – with fictitious names – arising from the reflective practice used throughout the Sheffield project. They illustrate how the liturgical methods have a profound effect for individuals, and are divided into four sections:

The valuing of individuals and building of community

The community, which includes residents, care staff, relatives and sometimes children, is built up and individuals are respected:

---

5 L. W. Howard, *Using Godly Play with Alzheimer's and Dementia Patients*, Morehouse Education Resource, 2015, resource available at www.churchpublishing.org/products/usinggodlyplaywithalzheimers anddementiapatients.

Setting 1

The care staff and the residents of a care setting for independent living were having difficulty with the way Arthur, who has dementia, was responding to them. It was observed that the Godly Play sessions allowed Arthur to work well in community. The individual welcome given to each person and the building of the circle meant that Arthur felt valued and therefore accepted the request of the storyteller to let others have a turn at speaking, whereas in other situations this would have resulted in confrontation.[6]

Setting 2

Every Wednesday morning 16 pre-schoolers marched in and sat at the feet of the 'Grandmas' and 'Grandpas' for a Godly Play story. [They] would wonder together after the story and then sing together. Finally the children would give hugs to all the 'Grandmas' and 'Grandpas'. This was the highlight of the week for both the children and the older adults. For some of the Alzheimer's folks it was the only time in the week that they smiled.[7]

Reminiscence

Reminiscence can take place during any part of the liturgy:

Setting 3

Godly Play was tried out in a Bible study for Spanish-speaking people with early stage Alzheimer's disease and found to be tremendously successful. One Christmas, for example, one participant responded to the 'I wonder' questions by reciting

---

6 I am indebted to my colleague Kathryn Lord for Settings 1 and also 4 to 11.

7 Setting 2 is from Howard, *Godly Play*, p. 12.

a poem she had learned when she was a child. Another woman told us that Fidel Castro took Christmas away from them in Cuba. She then described Cuba without Christmas as if it had just happened yesterday. During the telling of the Creation story participants energetically echoed my words every time I said, 'And God saw that it was good.' The programme kept people engaged and helped them recover lost memories.[8]

Setting 4

Each person in the group is given a 'Wellbeing box' in which they can store objects that are special to them, including from their life story and from the Godly Play stories. The sensory stimulation helps them – during the individual Response Time – to access memories of their own story as well as the Christian story. The Wellbeing boxes are given to everyone in the session, including carers, so that the people with dementia are not singled out and so that all take part. This is spiritual wellbeing for everyone.

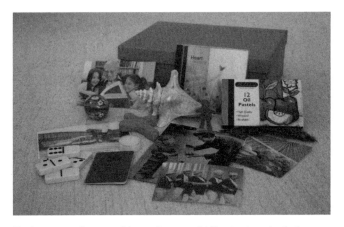

Each person chooses objects they would like to store in their 'Wellbeing box'

8 Cited on Facebook.

Mental and spiritual health support

Godly Play leads to discovery and meaning-making – both verbally and non-verbally – by allowing time for reflection. The older people with dementia are affirmed, esteemed and valued:

Setting 5

Because the participants had been able to enter into the story of Holy Week – which was told using a beautiful wooden model of Jerusalem – this enabled a deep reflection about the washing of feet and the cross. A visiting sister had joined us and, whilst holding the hand of her brother who has dementia, wondered with the group about grace, love and forgiveness in family relationships.

Setting 6

During the Response Time people were given the choice as to what object they wanted to hold. Dora held a compact mirror and chatted to a member of the team about how at 80 years old she had written an article for a newspaper on fashion for older women. The conversation and mood then shifted, as it often does with Dora, when she began to focus on the mistakes she had made in life. The team member suggested that they both look into the mirror and say to themselves, and to each other – 'You are a beautiful person'. They laughed great big belly laughs as they did this.

Setting 7

Barbara laid out the Ten Commandments from the story and a large shell on a coffee table and spent half an hour drawing the shell and writing some commandments inside and around a big heart. She was pleased with her finished picture – 'Do not covet what others have' was written out three times along with a new commandment, 'Honour yourself'. She explained that she no longer has parents and so had written a new commandment.

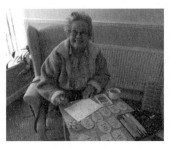 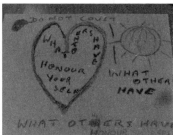

Barbara responding to the story of the Ten Commandments

Maintaining self and purpose

The strengths, passions and abilities of the older people are followed, and they are enabled to bless one another in liturgy that is fully participatory:

Setting 8

During the Response Time a lady was telling the storyteller how she used to sing in her church choir but felt increasingly excluded from the congregation. Together they quietly practised singing 'Praise God from whom all blessings flow' and the lady was surprised at how the tune just came to her. At the final blessing this lady beautifully led the group in the singing.

Setting 9

After the story of the Ten Commandments Alice (who has very poor hearing and sight) arranged the tree blocks to mirror the way the story had been set out. Alice showed off her creation with a beaming smile, thinking back to the time when her teacher had told her that she was 'no good at art'.

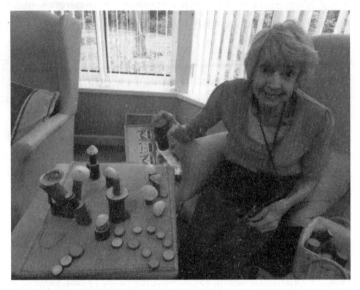

Alice with her arrangements of the tree blocks as the Ten Commandments

Setting 10

During the Response Time Edna chose to write out John 3.16 ('For God so loved the world . . .') and was pleased to read these words out to everyone during the Feast.

Setting 11

Performing an act of loving service to the group by always volunteering to wash up after the Feast was very important to Sheila who was the wife of a retired minister.

International links and collaboration with others

The sharing of reflective practice stories from around the world (Europe, Australia and the USA) allows for an evolving and exciting innovation in liturgical action using Godly Play for people with dementia. A chapter on how to adapt the method for use with older people (including those who are living with dementia) in the book *Godly Play – European Perspectives on Practice and Research* is leading to wider communication.[9]

The project has made presentations at the Research Symposium on Ageing and Spirituality (March 2017 and March 2018) and at the New Contextual Church Conference (April 2018). There is collaboration with others interested in this field of work: writing articles for the Christian Council on Ageing; working together with a trainer for Playlist for Life; joining forces with Livability to organize a conference on creative approaches to dementia; and presenting workshops at Care Home Roadshows and at several Anglican and Methodist workshops on ministry with older people. The Advisory Group for Stories for the Soul includes academics working in the fields of gerontology, occupational therapy, chaplaincy and sociological studies.

The challenges and the work ahead

Challenges of the Godly Play sessions include: adapting the story materials so people with dementia and people with visual and hearing impairment can engage their senses and access the story; adapting the choices in the Response Time so they are appropriate for people with dementia; enabling the older people to serve one another safely in the 'Feast' time. The varied nature of the needs of people with dementia and the

---

9 M. Steinhauser and R. Oystese, *Godly Play – European Perspectives on Practice and Research*, Münster: Waxmann, 2018.

uniqueness of each group means there is no 'one size fits all'. Our method is to develop support and training materials and to suggest a variety of best possible practices that those at local level can draw from and adapt to their unique situation.

The words 'Godly' and 'Play' can be misunderstood and are a barrier to care staff, to older people and to their relatives, and for this reason the sessions can be helpfully renamed 'Stories for the Soul'. A website, www.storiesforthesoul.org, was launched to communicate to care settings and to Christians involved in ministry among people with dementia the benefits that Godly Play can bring. There are many challenges in under-resourced care settings for staff to be liberated to support our voluntary sessions effectively and there are financial and time challenges for churches and volunteers of sustaining this ministry of spiritual care.

To lead Godly Play sessions well it is highly recommended that people attend the three-day accredited course provided by Godly Play UK: the investment of time and money for the training and resources can sometimes be an obstacle. It is encouraging that from the three diverse care settings that have been worked most closely with in Sheffield, three employees have chosen to train as spiritual accompaniers in Godly Play: a chaplain for the Methodist Homes Association, an activities co-ordinator and a mental health nurse.

The liturgical integrity of Godly Play demonstrates that there are different ways to approach community life together – for employees and residents and relatives and other visitors including volunteers themselves, and there is the potential for this to help bring a change in the culture of care. An adaptation of Godly Play – called Deep Talk – for use in secular settings may prove effective for the training of care staff to understand the ethos of this method and to enable them to think through purpose, value, hope and meaning in their workplace. Deep Talk may also prove beneficial for older people who may have no religious background but would benefit from such a story-based participatory method.

The Godly Play session ends with a 'Feast'. A new communion for people living with dementia, which also uses some of the verbal and non-verbal language of Godly Play, is being developed and would be a very valuable addition to the liturgy of Stories for the Soul.

CASE STUDY 3: MESSY VINTAGE IN JERSEY
(Written with Katie Norman)

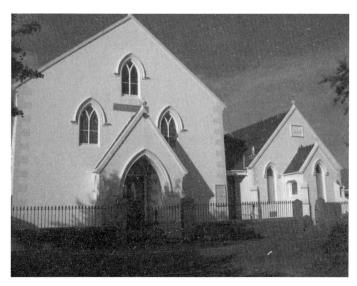

Philadelphie Messy Centre

Messy Vintage was brought to life in a Methodist church in Jersey and forms part of a remarkable story of faith expressed by a small ageing congregation in a rural area of the Channel Islands.

Messy Church

Messy Church is a fun way of being church for families. It is designed for all ages, is based on creativity, hospitality and celebration, and is part of the Bible Reading Fellowship. There are nearly 4,000 Messy Churches in 39 countries around the world. Messy Church builds relationships with people outside the church context, providing creative resources to engage people who don't already belong to another form of church. It typically includes a welcome, a long creative time to explore the biblical theme through getting messy; a short celebration time involving story, prayer, song, games and similar; and a sit-down meal together at tables. All elements are for, and should include, people of all ages, adults and children. Most Messy Churches meet once a month. It models good ways of growing as a family.

Seeds sown

Katie Norman, national co-ordinator for Messy Vintage, was intrigued when she first heard about Messy Church and longed for it to come to Jersey. For two years she prayed earnestly that a way would be found, little thinking she would become the answer to her own prayers. She spent ten years of her working life in primary education but did not consider herself a 'crafty person'. A local preacher in the Methodist Circuit, Philadelphie Methodist had been her church family all her life, but its congregation was dwindling in size and getting older, so that it was proving difficult to find volunteers to step into the role of steward. When a new minister's first question to Katie was 'Have you heard of Messy Church?' she had a dawning sense that God might be asking her to begin Messy Church in Jersey.

The work at Philadelphie began with Messy Church for families in the usual format, but Katie started noticing how all-age worship engaged members of the congregation from a local care home for people with special needs: 'They came alive. People who struggled to converse were clearly worshipping.' This gave her the idea of offering Messy Church to adults, including those with learning disabilities and dementia. With the full backing of her minister, the Revd Christine Legge, the two of them swiftly put things in place and Philadelphie began monthly Messy Vintage sessions in 2011. Soon after, Messy Vintage was taken 'on the road' to the first care home.

A radical decision

Messy Church outgrew Philadelphie's capacity to host. The pews were a hindrance to expanding and the seeds of a radical plan began to germinate in the congregation and within the Methodist Circuit. Why not take out the pews and turn the entire space into a Messy Church? Sunday services would end, and instead the focus would be all things Messy. With some trepidation the idea was presented to the congregation and the decision to take this bold step was reached unanimously. The final Sunday service was held in December 2012. Following a period of renovation, the building reopened as Philadelphie Messy Church in February 2013. It is now known as Philadelphie Messy Centre. On Sundays, members of the congregation now worship at Bethlehem Methodist Church, which has enthusiastically supported the development of its neighbour's new Messy ministry.

Co-ordinating a growing team

Katie has a dedicated team of 28 volunteers committed to seeing Messy Vintage reaching as many older people in their local community as possible. The project is labour-intensive, and each volunteer fulfils a vital role. There is a deep sense of fellowship and mission in the ecumenical team, which unites its members. Some team members were on the edges of church life when Philadelphie functioned as a traditional Methodist place of worship; now they are fully engaged. Nurturing this team and co-ordinating its activity is a huge undertaking. Each month Messy Vintage is held at the Messy Centre in Philadelphie, and Messy Vintage on the Road is taken to five care settings. The dates and times for these 72 sessions are published at the beginning of the year, and each one must be resourced with volunteers and craft supplies. Themes are set in advance and there is a monthly planning meeting. The team have regular retreats where they laugh, share and grow together. Katie says the team are a great blessing and it has been essential to have the right team and to value each member. 'They are amazing!'

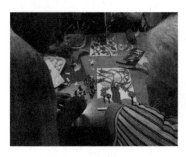 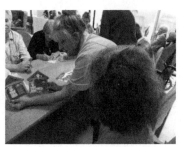

Messy Vintage on the Road

Craft activities linking to a theme

The common element in each session, which makes it 'Messy', is the craft activity. Of the 12 sample sessions you can download from the 'Gift of Years' website, session 6 is entitled 'Messy Harvest', based on the parable of the growing seed (Mark 4.26–29). The craft described is to create a scarecrow, whose role is to watch over the crops as they grow. Scarecrow-making materials are listed as: thin garden canes; green garden tape; round polystyrene balls; cupcake cases; wood; eyes; peppercorns; raffia; material; ribbon; funky foam or material scraps; scissors; double-sided sticky tape or glue stick.

While the craft is happening, with much support from volunteers, conversation is encouraged around the theme, drawing on childhood memories and life experiences. Laughter and sharing are regular features. Introducing the theme through the craft activity means that, when the next part of the session arrives, where the theme is addressed by the session leader, members of the group have already been introduced to the topic.

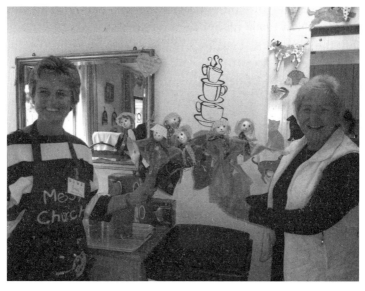

Scarecrows made during a 'Messy Harvest' session

Celebration expanding on the theme

Moving into the part of the session that is called the Celebration, the leader builds on the discussions that have already started through the craft activity. For the 'Messy Harvest' session, Jesus' parable about the growing seed is retold and a story shared from the leader's life about feeling watched over and protected, which leads to reflection on God's ever-present watchful love for each person. The leader might bring in seed-lings and explain what they have come from and what they might become, and how they need nurturing.

A time of singing Christian songs is included towards the end of each session. Katie says that recorded music works well if there are no musicians to play. She uses *Hymns We Have Loved* and takes in large-print copies of the booklet that goes with the three CDs. Music chosen draws from the songs that par-ticipants will have sung in their younger years. For the Messy Harvest session, this might include: 'We plough the fields and scatter'; 'Now thank we all our God'; 'Great is thy faithfulness'; 'For the fruits of his creation'. Katie reflects that upbeat songs also work well with the groups. Even in end-of-life care set-tings, where people are weak and frail, participants respond to the rhythm of a lively song. A blend of traditional music to spark memories, and contemporary songs to enliven the group, seems to work well.

Every session has a time of prayer for others, with members of the group invited to share people and situations for which they would like prayer. There is time for the traditional version of the Lord's Prayer, which is known by almost everyone, and the sessions finish with a Messy Vintage version of The Grace with actions:

May the grace of our Lord Jesus Christ
(Hold out your hands as if expecting a present)
And the love of God
(Put your hands on your heart)
And the fellowship of the Holy Spirit
(Hands outstretched)
Be with us all, now and forever.
(Look around and bless each other)
Amen!

5

Dementia-friendly Churches

DAVID RICHARDSON

'You shall not revile the deaf or put a stumbling-block before the blind; you shall fear your God; I am the LORD' (Leviticus 19.14). These are perhaps the earliest words in world literature to underscore the importance of sensitivity towards the needs of people with disabilities. They are of course given added force by being set within the context of obedience to God. One of the particular challenges that the Church faces today is that of being responsive to the needs of people affected by dementia – and of doing so in the context of worship of God and of service to the world that Christ came to save.

There are two terms that will recur in this chapter, and for which the following definitions might assist:

- 'Dementia-friendly': this means aware of, and responsive to, the interests and needs of people affected by dementia.
- 'People affected by dementia': this embraces not just those who have been diagnosed with the condition, but also their carer – if they have one – and other close family members and friends.

What is a 'dementia-friendly church'? According to Dr Elizabeth Anderson, a dementia adviser in the Diocese of Leeds, it is a church

- that is welcoming and inclusive towards people with dementia and their carers;

- where the church leadership and other members of the congregation help people with dementia to feel safe and oriented within the church environment;
- where it is OK to get confused and forget things;
- where people with dementia and their carers feel that they are valued members of the congregation, stay involved in church activity, and do not 'fall off the radar'.

This chapter offers advice as to how a church might become dementia-friendly. It reports in some detail on one current project, involving the use of local volunteers ('Dementia Enablers') across a broad spectrum of denominations and spanning the whole county of Cumbria.

There is one issue of language to be faced at the outset. The term 'dementia sufferer' should be avoided. 'People living with dementia' stresses the fact that those who have received the diagnosis may continue to make their own decisions and to live life the way they would wish. By doing so, they give heart to others and help to dispel myths and combat prejudice. That the latter stages of the dementia journey may be beset by difficulty is not denied. The Church should see the picture as a whole and ensure that the love of God is made clear – in good times, in bad times, and all the time.

The challenge of dementia

To begin, a church needs to address the scale of the challenge. Dementia is not an issue that simply causes memory problems for a few old people – and thus something that, while it may be distressing for those immediately involved, need not perhaps be of concern to the rest of us.

Dementia is about more than memory: it can adversely affect an individual's ability to communicate and undertake everyday tasks. The following extract from a *Times* leader expresses it well:

Alzheimer's is a relentless thief of individual autonomy. Missed hospital appointments and keys left in strange places give way to more crippling incapacities. Ordinary tasks like going to the shops for a pint of milk can become insuperable obstacles to getting through the day or, worse, fraught with risk. Yet just as a sufferer's self-sufficiency recedes, so friends and acquaintances sometimes drift away, repelled by the stigma of the disease or uncertain how to react to its vicissitudes.[1]

I will overlook the use of the word 'sufferer' in the extract.

Dementia takes many forms (there are in fact over 100 of them, including combinations involving more than one form). The most common are:

- *Alzheimer's disease* – sometimes used as a synonym for dementia – is the most prevalent form. During the course of the disease, proteins build up in the brain to form structures called 'plaques' and 'tangles'. This leads to the loss of connections between nerve cells, and eventually to the death of nerve cells and loss of brain tissue.
- *Vascular dementia* – the second most common form – is caused by reduced blood supply to the brain due to diseased blood vessels.

The other types of dementia include:

- *Dementia with Lewy bodies* – tiny spherical structures develop inside nerve cells, and symptoms often include fluctuating alertness, hallucinations and problems with movement.
- *Frontotemporal dementia* – damage occurs first in the front and side of the brain; personality, behaviour or language are initially more affected than memory.

---

1 'Illness and independence', *The Times*, 28 December 2017, www.thetimes.co.uk/article/illness-and-independence-50h9wzb5x.

There are currently estimated to be 850,000 people with dementia in the UK. This number is set to rise to over a million by 2021 and two million by the middle of the twenty-first century. The figure of two million is equivalent to one in four of the present population of Greater London or four times the population of Cumbria. At any one time up to a quarter of all hospital beds are occupied by people with dementia (who have, in most instances, been admitted for treatment of other conditions). It has been estimated that, within the average general practice, the number of people likely to develop dementia is the same as the number of women likely to become pregnant.

The cost of dementia (in terms of its impact on health and social care, the economy and individuals and their families) is estimated at £25.3 billion per year – enough to pay the energy bill for every household in the UK for a year. Dementia is not just a condition affecting those of older age. There are 42,000 people with dementia under the age of 65. The decline associated with early-onset dementia may be more rapid than for people who develop dementia at a later age. Just over 7 per cent of those aged over 65 have dementia. A person's risk of developing it increases from 1 in 14 between the ages of 65 and 69 to 1 in 6 over the age of 80.

Dementia is a problem not just for one country but for the whole planet. It affects almost 50 million people at the moment; the rate of increase equates to one new case every 3.2 seconds (1,125 an hour). By 2050 there will be 131.5 million living with dementia, with over two-thirds of them living in low- and middle-income countries. The cost of dementia worldwide is estimated to be $1 trillion a year.

Dementia is at present incurable. There are some treatments that can slow down the pace of Alzheimer's, but they only work for a limited period, and they cannot reverse or halt the disease. The amount of money spent on dementia research in the UK is about one-eighth of that allocated for cancer.

Taking steps to become dementia-friendly

A church that wishes to be dementia-friendly needs to identify the specific actions that it will take. There are, however, two counter-arguments that may need rebuttal first.

The first is that the matter is already in hand: 'While members applauded all that was being done to raise awareness of the needs of those affected by dementia, they felt that those needs were already being sensitively taken care of. They didn't feel, therefore, that having someone with a particular responsibility in this area would add anything to what is already happening in the church.' The above and following quotations are from the response of a parochial church council invited to participate in the Cumbria project. The second argument stems from the view that 'there are lots of other conditions we should be thinking about as well. We can't concentrate on just one.'

The answer to the first is that what is assumed to be everyone's concern may end up as nobody's responsibility. The second may be answered by reference to the particular needs of people with dementia and those who care for them, and also by the fact that whatever makes a church dementia-friendly will be of benefit to the congregation more generally.

One key step is to designate a member of the church who will take a lead on dementia matters, which might include the appointment of

- a chaplain (or similar) who will have immediate or particular pastoral responsibility for people affected by dementia;
- someone who will encourage the church as a whole to become dementia-friendly.

These two options are of course not incompatible with each other.

The Cumbria project follows the second option. The project was launched by Churches Together in Cumbria (CTiC) in 2015 with the aim of 'making every church in Cumbria dementia-friendly by 2020'. It is worth remarking that this is one area where churches can work constructively and harmoniously together. Dementia is no respecter of denominational boundaries.

CTiC appointed a Dementia Coordinator (the author of this chapter) and established a Dementia Reference Group to work with him. The members of the Group were drawn from six of CTiC's member denominations. They are a mix of clerical and lay; all have had professional or personal engagement with dementia, and one is also the county volunteer representative for Alzheimer's Society. It was, however, recognized from the start that the project would only prosper if there was specific, local commitment. A distinctive title was sought, and 'Dementia Enabler' was coined as descriptor for the local volunteer. The following were identified as the key components of the role. It was agreed that the Enabler

- should be, or become, a Dementia Friend and should encourage others to become Dementia Friends also;
- should have a general awareness of the support services that are available in their local community for people affected by dementia;
- should encourage the local church or group of churches to become dementia-friendly (in terms of welcome, worship and environment).

'Dementia Friend' refers to an Alzheimer's Society programme. This 'is the biggest ever initiative to change people's perceptions of dementia. It aims to transform the way the nation thinks, acts and talks about the condition.' People become Friends by attending a one-hour information session or by enrolling online:

A Dementia Friend learns a little bit more about what it's like to live with dementia and then turns that understanding into action – anyone of any age can be a Dementia Friend ... Being a Dementia Friend simply means learning more about dementia, putting yourself in the shoes of someone living with the condition, and turning your understanding into action. From visiting someone you know with dementia to being more patient in a shop queue, every action counts.

The information session seeks to dispel some of the myths surrounding dementia, such as 'it's a natural part of ageing', to make people look at those with the condition in a new light ('there's more to a person than the dementia') and to encourage them to take some action that will make life that bit better for someone with the condition.

There are currently over 2.3 million Dementia Friends across the country, the target being 4 million by 2020. Information sessions are delivered by Dementia Friends Champions and it is encouraging to note that several Enablers have gone on to become Champions and are thus now able to lead sessions in their own churches and elsewhere.

'General awareness of the support services' refers to that which is on offer within the county from Age UK, Alzheimer's Society and other charities, and from the memory service of the Cumbria Partnership NHS Trust. Inclusion of this is not meant to imply that the Enabler is to be the local expert on all dementia-related questions – but it does recognize the fact that people may well, and rightly, see them as an initial port of call. Signposting to such services is provided in CTiC's 'Dementia Enablers' Handbook'.

Being a Dementia Friend and having knowledge of local services provide a necessary backdrop to the most important of the three elements: 'encourage the local church to become dementia-friendly, in terms of welcome, worship and environment'. These points may be summarized as 'how', 'what' and 'where':

- *How* do we communicate with people with dementia and their carers; how do we make people welcome?
- *What* steps can we take to help people with dementia take part in worship? What might dementia-friendly worship entail?
- *Where* can we (within the constraints of a given place of worship) ensure that it is accessible for people with dementia and that issues such as safety, signage, use of space and lighting are addressed?

Local churches were asked not just to identify a Dementia Enabler but also formally to nominate them for that role. A familiar feature of many churches is the person who is an enthusiast for a cause that lies close to their heart, but that rarely surfaces in the mind of anyone else except perhaps at an annual coffee morning. We were determined not to allow it to appear that this was such a venture.

The nomination form is signed by the minister or other church leader, and reads:

> I hereby declare on behalf of the [Name of church or group of churches] that we will play our part in seeking to make every church in Cumbria dementia-friendly by 2020. Specifically, we hereby nominate [Name] to serve as Dementia Enabler for the said church or group of churches. We undertake that we will support the Dementia Enabler:
>
> - By our prayers.
> - By giving them opportunity to report regularly to the church council or other appropriate body.
> - By giving due consideration to their recommendations as to ways in which we may become dementia-friendly.
> - By meeting such agreed expenses as they may reasonably incur in fulfilling their responsibilities.

We think it important that the office of Enabler be regarded as on a par with other offices – by, for example, the holder being named on the inside front cover of the church magazine or on the weekly notice sheet.

We do not leave the Dementia Enablers comfortless. We provide a monthly e-newsletter; this includes a list of the places of worship where there is an Enabler, updated as new ones are appointed, and includes the name and email address of the Enabler where they have agreed to be identified in this way. There is an annual county-wide 'Development Day' for Enablers, supplemented by periodic local fellowship meetings, in recognition of the difficulty of getting people together in a county that is 60 miles long by 45 miles wide. To date, 110

Dementia Enablers have been recruited, covering over 150 churches, chapels and other places of worship. Some of them have two, most have one, and in some instances an Enabler is responsible for a whole circuit or benefice. The denominations currently involved are: the Church of England, the Church of Scotland, the Roman Catholic Church, the Baptist, Methodist and United Reformed Churches, the King's Church, the Salvation Army and the Society of Friends.

The necessary first step towards making the local church more dementia-friendly is to take a critical look at things as they now are, in terms of the 'how', 'what' and 'where'. In this context we have been much helped by staff of the charity Livability who devised a questionnaire for us. Dementia Enablers were asked to consider the following in respect of the congregation:

Are you aware of:

- anyone in your congregation who is affected by dementia?
- anyone showing possible early signs of dementia such as confusion, forgetfulness or difficulty in communicating?
- someone who has had the diagnosis, still living at home or now in residential care?
- someone caring for a spouse or family member still at home or who is now in residential care?
- someone caring for a family member who lives some distance away?
- someone keeping an eye on a friend or neighbour with dementia (or regularly visiting a friend or neighbour who is now in residential care)?
- any children or young people under 18 who have someone with dementia in their immediate family (or who have a family member caring for someone with dementia)?
- anyone who has developed early-onset dementia?

The above serves to dispel any lingering sense that the impact of dementia is restricted to a few elderly people.

We then asked how many of the following still attend church services, or church groups or activities on a regular basis:

- People with dementia living at home?
- People with dementia in residential care?
- Family carers?

With some idea of numbers involved one was then able to consider the physical environment – with reference to seeing, hearing, comfort and safety. Questions to be addressed included:

- How well lit are the toilets?
- How clear are the signs to the toilet doors?
- How clear are the notice boards?
- Does the church have a hearing loop (and is it turned on)?
- Does everyone involved in leading the service use a microphone?
- How warm is your church, especially on cold days?
- How open are the congregation to allowing people with dementia to walk around if they need to?
- How much quiet space do you have if people with dementia need to leave the service for any reason?
- How uneven are the paths and grounds around your church?
- How frayed are your carpets?
- How easy is it to get to the front for communion (are there steps or other obstacles to negotiate)?

This may serve to underscore the point that the aspects that are designed with the needs of people with dementia foremost will also serve to the advantage of people more generally. We would all, for instance, benefit from smoother paths, better-lit toilets and safer carpets.

These considerations provide the backdrop for addressing the pastoral engagement of the church:

- If the church has a pastoral ministry team, do its members visit people with dementia in their own homes or care homes; is there any specific support for carers?
- Does the church take the needs of people with dementia into account in planning or delivering services?
- Does the church understand what those needs are?
- Does the church conduct worship in residential homes, involving people with dementia?
- Has anyone been trained to lead dementia-friendly worship?

No church should be isolated from its local community, and the questionnaire invited consideration first of local provision for people affected by dementia and then of the church's links thereto:

- Is your area recognized as a dementia-friendly community?
- Which dementia charities work in your area?
- Are there any community projects that support people with dementia?
- Are there any residential care homes that specialize in dementia care?
- Are there any local carer support groups?
- What links does the church – whether the minister, the pastoral team, or people affected by dementia or other members – have to relevant community organizations?
- What links does the church have to residential care homes?

The questionnaire concluded with three questions:

1 How important is it to work towards becoming a dementia-friendly church (on a spectrum from 'we need to make a start' through 'we are doing OK but need to do more' to 'we are already dementia-friendly')?
2 How open is the church (including the minister) to becoming dementia-friendly (on a spectrum from 'not very open' to 'ready to go')?
3 If the church is already dementia-friendly, is there more that it could do?

There are, of course, no right or wrong answers. What was sought is an honest appraisal of 'things as they are', rather than things as ideally they might be. Also, the form was not to be completed by the Enabler on their own. It provided opportunity to secure early engagement from the minister and lay leaders.

The training offered to Enablers was spread over two days – an initial morning event which included a Dementia Friends session (needed for those who had not previously attended one, and serving as a refresher for those who had), followed several weeks later by a day-long conference at which they were asked to reflect on what they had learnt through the questionnaire.

The changes wrought by the project may be characterized both as quantifiable and unquantifiable. The latter relates to the adoption of new or more sensitive attitudes on the part of church leaders because of the quiet lobbying of the Dementia Enabler, and the greater involvement of members of the congregation in making and maintaining contact with people with dementia and their carers – for example, making them welcome at church and visiting them at home or in a care home.

Some of the quantifiable changes are summarized as:

- The introduction of regular 'Tea Services' (short, dementia-friendly acts of worship, followed by tea and cake) at a number of locations across the county – six at the moment of writing, but with more planned.
- The preparation of dementia-friendly pew cards in one rural benefice.
- The organizing of a 'dementia tea' but with a fun and friendly music theme ('sort of old time music hall with a Christian message') – by invitation only 'so as not to overcrowd the hall and so that it might be locals who may well recognize each other'.
- The holding of a cathedral service to mark Dementia Awareness Week.
- The establishment of a Memory Club, sponsored by the local Churches Together grouping.

- The introduction of a monthly support group called 'Minds in Tune' at one church.

There is one fact that should be recognized in this context – namely, that the long-term memory of a person with dementia may be more secure than the short-term one. The importance of familiar hymns, of the Authorized Version of the Bible and of the Book of Common Prayer (or other like manuals) cannot be over-emphasized.

A church can have a part to play in making the wider local community dementia-friendly. Its members may also take on a campaigning role – with a view, for example, to securing more training and support for family carers or an increase in the proportion of time given to dementia in the initial training of doctors and other health professionals.

Listening to people with dementia

To be truly dementia-friendly, the church will listen to, and be guided by, people who have received the diagnosis of dementia. It would do well to heed the words and catch the tone of the statements in the five bullet points below. They have been issued by Alzheimer's Society but 'reflect the things people with dementia have said are essential to their quality of life. Grounded in human rights law, they are a rallying call to improve the lives of people with dementia and to recognize that they shouldn't be treated differently because of their diagnosis':

- We have the right to be recognized as who we are, to make choices about our lives including taking risks, and to contribute to society. Our diagnosis should not define us, nor should we be ashamed of it.
- We have the right to continue with day-to-day and family life, without discrimination or unfair cost, to be accepted and included in our communities and not live in isolation or loneliness.

- We have the right to an early and accurate diagnosis, and to receive evidence-based, appropriate, compassionate and properly funded care and treatment, from trained people who understand us and how dementia affects us. This must meet our needs, wherever we live.
- We have the right to be respected, and recognized as partners in care, provided with education, support, services, and training that enables us to plan and make decisions about the future.
- We have the right to know about, and decide if we want to be involved in, research that looks at cause, cure and care for dementia and be supported to take part.

These statements provide a yardstick against which the changes in attitude that a church is seeking to inculcate might be measured.

Guidance as to the specific actions that a church might take may be found in a study undertaken by Julia Burton-Jones (Dementia Specialist Project Officer for the Diocese of Rochester). In the following section, the quotes are the comments of people with dementia, and are followed by suggestions for action.

The importance of understanding and acceptance must be stressed.

'If friends at church have an awareness of the challenges dementia brings, they will respond with kindness and sensitivity. They will not mind if brain changes make me say or do unusual things. They will make allowances and accommodate my disability.'

Two ways in which we can help address this are:

- Dementia Friends' awareness sessions in churches.
- Learning alongside carers and people with dementia.

It is important, too, to ensure that people with dementia are included and valued, not overlooked and forgotten:

* * *

'Friends often struggle to cope with dementia and disappear. I need church to be a place where people are happy to see me and recognize I still have something to offer. It is hurtful when friends appear to be avoiding me.'

The ways we can help with this are:

- Remembering people with dementia in prayer.
- Welcoming and 'buddying' at services.
- Thinking through small group structures and having alternatives for those who struggle with thinking tasks.

But there is more to life than church! There is a need for friendship to combat the fact or the risk of isolation:

* * *

'Opportunities to socialize are important in keeping me independent and helping me enjoy life. Social activities at church are stimulating and a great source of friendship.'

It is important that we should make sure that all church social activities are inclusive, and that we should also offer regular or occasional activities aimed at those with dementia. We can also support local organizations providing groups – for example, through discounted use of halls, help with publicity or providing volunteers.

People with dementia may need appropriate spiritual support.

* * *

'Conventional services are less easy as they demand concentration and cognitive abilities, but my faith is still important to me. Pastoral support at the right level will allow my faith to continue to nurture and sustain me.'

Here a mix of answers may be appropriate. We should maintain some services that follow familiar patterns. We should offer occasional memory-friendly services. We should pray and worship with care-home residents with dementia and visit those still in their own homes. We should not forget the spiritual needs of the carer and should seek to ensure that they themselves are able to continue attending church.

All this may avail nothing without practical help.

* * *

'Simple practical support can make a big difference. A friend from church might pop round for an hour or two to keep me company so that my carer can go out. We might also value help with transport and shopping.'

Practical help might include:

- Suggesting a regular time when you can be with the person with dementia, providing friendship and giving the carer a short break.
- Offering help with transport.

People may need help coping with difficult feelings and changing relationships.

* * *

'Dementia can cause painful reactions because of the way it changes life and relationships. Someone willing to listen and allow me to tell my story can relieve the stress.'

Some of the answers might be:

• Keeping in touch through visits, phone calls, emails or texts.
• Practising active listening.
• Advertising local support groups and helplines of organizations supporting people with dementia (such as, but not limited to, Age UK and Alzheimer's Society).

The comments offered above, and the actions proposed in response, give an invaluable checklist against which a church can compare its own activity.

The challenge for the churches

There are a number of obstacles that may lie in the path for a church seeking to become and remain dementia-friendly. One awkward truth to be faced is that churches operate within a society that does not hold the elderly in high regard. This may readily be illustrated. With the statistic in mind that 1 in 6 of the population over 80 is likely to develop dementia, one can imagine the outcry there would be if there were a condition that affected, say, 18 per cent of teenage boys or a similar percentage of women of child-bearing age, and if it were disclosed that there was no cure and that research into the condition was significantly underfunded. But because dementia principally affects the elderly, society does not make any comparable fuss.

While few would actually deny the importance of ministry to the elderly, it lies under the shadow of 'and'. The word is both a conjunction and a qualifier, in that what comes after it is thereby stated to be less important than what comes before. A local church's mission action plan may indicate an ambition to increase its outreach to 'schools and care homes' – and that will win praise as indicating an even-handed approach to ministry.

Were the formulation to be 'care homes and schools', it would come across as having its priorities wrong. A church may need reminding that Jesus told Peter not just to 'feed my lambs' but to 'feed my sheep'!

Those who are uneasy about any focus on ministry to the elderly (whether they believe that outreach to the young should have priority or – frankly – because they do not wish to contemplate themselves becoming old) might be reminded that dementia casts its shadow across the generations.

Let us meet Jane. She is an active member of her local church. She is in her mid-forties. Her career is prospering, the pay is good, and there are hints of a major promotion soon – but there are problems. Her husband's job is far from secure, her 11-year-old is unhappy at 'big school' and her 16-year-old daughter is embodying the stereotypical sulky teenager. Jane gets a phone call from her father: 'I am really worried about your mother. She is getting very forgetful and when we were out in the car the other day she would have gone the wrong way around a roundabout if I had not been with her. Can you please come and see us?' And Jane thinks: 'Why, Lord, why me, why now? Can't my useless brother and my selfish sister-in-law do something to help? They live so much closer. I don't have time. I have to see Luke's form tutor, I am running Messy Church on Saturday, and I am doing the intercessions on Sunday morning.'

Let us now meet Mark. He has always been close to his grandfather. When he was ten, Grandpa somehow managed to get hold of tickets for the two of them to go to Lord's for the test match the last time the Australians were here – but now something has changed. Grandpa has lost interest in cricket, he rarely goes out, he forgets things (including Mark's last birthday), and he has started calling Mark 'Ted' (and there has been no one of that name in the family since Grandpa's own Uncle Ted).

Dementia presents a challenge to faith. Of course, for those with no faith, dementia may prove their suspicion that there is no real purpose to life and that one simply must take one's chance with whatever may come along. For people who believe that there is a god, it may prove that 'his' or 'her' or 'its' view of us is not ultimately well-intentioned. I think of the bleak remark of a friend of mine: 'There's one thing you can say about dementia. It proves that the Man Upstairs will get you in the end.' The only answer to that is that this is not the deity from whom the Christian ethos draws its inspiration. Or to express the gospel in terms of that metaphor, the Man Upstairs came downstairs in Palestine 2,000 years ago; God is not a remote, uncaring force.

For those with faith, the awkward truth is that God cannot cure dementia. Such a statement may cause upset or outrage, but a moment's reflection will show that it is true. The only other explanation is that God could effect a cure, but chooses not to. Reports that someone has been cured of dementia are to be dismissed. They are the religious equivalent of urban myths; they lie within the circumference of anecdote but are beyond the perimeter of verification. The only explanation for the story – unless the truth has been stretched beyond its permitted tolerances – is that the person is enjoying a period of stability in which their dementia has been temporarily halted or that there was a misdiagnosis and they never had dementia in the first place. A god who could answer a prayer that dementia be cured, but chose not to, would not be the God revealed in Christ. 'His ways are not our ways' is not the card to play in this context. A deity who capriciously withheld a cure would lack common decency, let alone be the exemplar of human completeness found in Christ.

To state that God cannot cure dementia is not a denial of his power. It is, rather, to recognize that he works within the parameters of the world he made and came to save. I am writing this on a cold winter's afternoon in Cumbria. Much as I might wish, I cannot, by clicking my heels, be transported to a warm springtime morning in Cornwall. I am 74; I cannot, even if I wanted, become 47 again. A crop sown in March for an autumn harvest would not yield a crop in April, no matter how fervently the parish prayer chain might intercede. God can work miracles, but he does not do magic.

The question arises as to the relevance for people with dementia of 'prayers for healing'. It is important to ensure that everyone involved is aware that the word 'healing' is being used in a restricted way that does not accord with its everyday meaning. A grandchild who hears that the church is including Gran in its prayers for healing will have a perspective different from that of someone who has attended an invitation-only seminar on the topic. Prayers for a sense of peace for the person with dementia or for fortitude or resilience for a carer are valid and can be answered, but a church must be extremely careful not to appear to foster the misapprehension that a cure or a restoration to better health is in prospect.

Dementia may offer a particular challenge to those who have been accustomed to viewing life as micromanaged by God – most especially those who have espoused what is in effect a 'prosperity gospel', whereby today's temporary setback is but part of a divinely directed drama and will lead to tomorrow's greater opportunity. Such a gospel has its attractions as providing extra-terrestrial endorsement for the aspirations of the ambitious, healthy and comfortably circumstanced but is exposed as inadequate when one is faced with an incurable disease. Any attempt to reconcile such a view of God with the reality of dementia can lead to the most insensitive of remarks. Saying 'remember, God does not give us burdens greater than we can bear' may make the hearer think that 'if I (or my partner) were a weaker person, I (or they) would not have developed dementia'. Saying 'remember, everything happens for a purpose' may be heard as conveying the horrifying, unkind and wholly unchristian thought that it was the Lord's will that the person developed dementia.

Regrettably, one can still encounter people, even in church circles, who find something amusing in dementia. Saying to someone, 'I am going to an Alzheimer's Society coffee morning next week' can all too often evoke the reply, 'Don't forget to turn up!' Those who say such things would almost certainly not mock hearing loss or sight loss. Perhaps I might share a family reminiscence: my mother spent the last three and a half years of her life in a care home. On one occasion one of my sisters and I called to see her and took her out for lunch – to the café of a nearby garden centre. She looked around her and said, 'This is nice. Your dad would like it. Can we bring him next time?' This was a reasonable remark for the wife of a keen gardener to make. The only problem was that he had died two months earlier. She had been married for 64 years, and she could not remember that she had been bereaved.

This is not to deny a place to laughter – but humour must always be on the terms of people with dementia and not at their expense. Two true stories come to mind. One is of the couple living at home – the husband having dementia, and the wife being the carer. The parish priest comes to visit. The wife brings him into the house, opens the sitting room door, and says, 'Here's Father –', and her husband says, 'Christmas!' The second is of a lady living in a care home. The manager was doing the rounds in the dining room at breakfast. He bends over to ask her how she is. She seizes his tie, dangling over the cornflakes, and starts using it to polish her glasses. Few can resist a smile at the thought of the manager wholly at the mercy of the resident!

Remembering the carer

A dementia-friendly church will acknowledge the important part that the carer can play, whether that be a spouse or partner, or a family member or close friend. It may be a statement of the obvious but it bears repeating that not everyone with dementia has the support of a carer. The church should be alert to the estimate that one-third live domestically with a carer, another third are in residential care, and the final third live on their own. Women form the majority in this last category, given that their longevity tends to be greater than that of men.

Where there is a carer, the danger is of defining them by that role. The story in the Gospels of the healing of the daughter of the woman from Syrophoenicia may be instructive. At first reading, our Lord's apparent rejection of the mother's request ('it is not fair to take the children's food and throw it to the dogs') comes across as brutal and disrespectful. However, the promptness of her riposte ('yet even the dogs eat the crumbs that fall from their masters' table') shows that there was an element of banter to be read into the conversation. Jesus did not just see her – did not allow her to define herself – simply as the 'sick girl's mother'. She was a person in her own right, and he saw the need for her to have the chance to affirm her faith. The outcome was twofold – she received a treasured accolade ('woman, great is your faith') and 'her daughter was healed instantly'. If she went home with a smile on her face, as being the only person ever to get the better of God incarnate in repartee – then none of us would blame her!

It can be easy to stereotype the carer, not least by making three assumptions that may be correct but are not necessarily so.

One might assume that the carer has a real affection for the person with the diagnosis of dementia. Most do, of course, and see this as a challenge to be faced in the context of a life spent together. This attitude is exemplified by the husband who said: 'They always say that you should listen to experts. Well, we are the experts on Sally's dementia.' At the other end of the spectrum, I recall a man who visibly resented his wife's dementia – essentially because it stopped him doing the things that he had looked forward to in retirement. Fortunately, his displeasure was vented on the staff and volunteers of a local dementia support charity, and not on his wife.

One might possibly assume that the carer has a driving licence and is computer-literate. Invitations to a memory club (or a tea service) in a town three miles away, or a word of encouragement to download a page of helpful hints from this or that website, may be appreciated if these conditions are met, but will be felt to be insensitive if they are not. Furthermore, it might be assumed that the carer has no particular health problems of their own or other issues that concern them. This is almost certainly not true, given that they are probably in the later stages of their own life anyway, and is likely to become less true as the dementia takes its course and the needs of the person cared for increase.

The church should seek to ensure that the carer is both respected for the role that they play – for what may become a burden that they carry – and is also valued and loved for who they are themselves. Let us imagine starting a conversation with Jill, who is the carer for her husband Jack. Let the question 'How are you?' come across not as: 'I am just asking out of habit, and what I am really hoping is that you will tell me that Jack would not recognize me if I went to see him and so I don't need to feel bad for not doing so', but as: 'I am asking because I really care for you both, and I am going to go on visiting Jack, because I know it doesn't matter if he recognizes me or not. When I ask how you are, I do mean you-singular as well as you-plural. If you want to talk about Jack, that's fine. If you want to talk about anything other than Jack and his [expletive deleted] dementia, that's fine as well.'

The church will also need to be aware of the needs of those former carers whose loved ones have passed away. They may need the opportunity to talk, to unburden themselves of their experiences, but they will have unique insights that can both be of help to current carers, especially perhaps those embarking on that role, and can also guide the church as it seeks to become dementia-friendly. ('Former carer' is admittedly an awkward phrase. I recall one Alzheimer's Society branch that gracefully referred to them as the 'graduates' group'.)

The Church's commitment

I would in conclusion argue that the local church needs to demonstrate a medium-term and a long-term commitment if it is to be truly dementia-friendly. The former should take the form of a comprehensive and all-inclusive pledge to people affected by dementia. The story of Ruth and Naomi comes to mind (Ruth 1.16, 'Where you go, I will go; where you lodge, I will lodge'). Let our message echo that adamantine pledge:

We will be with you in the days when dementia may be no more than a cloud on a day of otherwise bright sunshine. We will be with you if the temperature drops and storms begin to gather. We will listen to you; we will seek your views. We will keep what you want us to keep and change what you need us to change. If you wish us to speak on your behalf we will do so boldly and gladly. We will make sure that all members of our churches understand about dementia. We will make you welcome at the services and at everything else. If the time comes when you cannot come to us we will come to you. Quite simply, we will never let go. We will make the church a beacon to the community, proclaiming that dementia is everybody's business and that anyone can do something to make a difference. We will seek to root out ignorance and stigma and insensitive behaviour wherever it may be found. We will honour family carers for what they do and will respect them as individuals. We will encourage those who provide care in whatever setting. We will support research and thus hasten the time when a cure is found and dementia is defeated. Until then we will echo Ruth: 'where you go, I will go; where you lodge, I will lodge' – even unto the end.

The long-term commitment must be to pray for a cure – to pray for a day when the statement that 'God cannot cure dementia' ceases to be true. Prayer needs to be practical, and to recognize that God will work his miracle through research, from which all may benefit, rather than the random halting of the condition in this or that patient.

Let us remember that effective prayer today for the recovery of cancer patients is facilitated by progress in research 20 or 30 years ago. 'God has no hands but our hands': these oft-quoted words of St Teresa of Avila might in this context be interpreted as 'God has no brain but our brains'. Let us see the search for a cure for dementia as a race between the ingenuity of the human brain and its frailty.

Prayer that ingenuity should win should be specific: for sufficient funding for research; for a flow of candidates willing to make a career in this field; for co-operation between institutions and across borders in dementia research; for co-operation between researchers and clinicians; and for patience and imagination on the part of all engaged in research.

Prayer should be frequent. There are certain topics that are likely to feature more often than others in a list of intercessions – such as the relief of poverty, the inculcation of a greater awareness of responsibility for the environment, and the plight of Christians persecuted for their faith or threatened with martyrdom. Let the cause of dementia research be included among them. Prayer should be accompanied by (other forms of) action – such as fundraising and the quiet word of encouragement to a science or medicine graduate to go into dementia research. They might be the person who makes the critical breakthrough.

In this chapter, I have sought to identify the scale of the problem, to dispel misunderstanding, to challenge myths and, above all, to show that a dementia-friendly church will be a positive place. It will show by its actions and its attitudes that 'dementia shall not have dominion'. It will – to echo Elizabeth Anderson's definition on pages 86–7 – be welcoming and inclusive towards people with dementia and their carers. It will help people with dementia to feel safe and oriented within the church environment. It will not mind if people get confused and forget things. It will encourage people to feel valued and stay involved, and it will never allow anyone to fall off the radar. It will care for carers. It will campaign with others to make the wider community dementia-friendly. By its activity today, and by its engagement with research for tomorrow, it will help hasten the time when the words of the Psalmist may come true (Psalm 91.5–6): 'You will not fear the terror of the night . . . or the pestilence that stalks in darkness'.

6

Music and Dementia:
Some Practical Considerations

SUE MOORE

The value of music for people with dementia

An increasing number of studies on the neurological function of those with differing forms of dementia point to some preservation of ability to recall familiar melodies and words of songs from earlier in life, and this is even more so in those individuals who have been practising musicians and/or who continue to play or sing after the onset of the condition. There is also some evidence that the practical skills of playing a musical instrument may be retained for a significant period after other skills have deteriorated. It is likely that learning and recall of music by playing (in particular) or singing (to a lesser extent) may make use of particular neural pathways that remain functional as dementia progresses.

Even where musical skills may not be fully retained in the long term, the role of music in improving emotional wellbeing in patients with dementia is demonstrable, and can encourage slightly longer-term retention of both verbal and visual memories. It has been suggested that participation in 'cognitive' leisure activities, including music, may be associated with a reduced risk of dementia, although further research is required to test this further.[1]

---

1 J. Verghese et al., 'Leisure activities and the risk of dementia in the elderly', *The New England Journal of Medicine* 348 (2003), pp. 2508–16.

Some studies[2] have also demonstrated improved recall of verbal information when sung rather than spoken, and one only has to think of the firmly imprinted words and melodies of children's nursery rhymes and playground songs to appreciate the longevity of songs learned in childhood. Music is often highly valued as a social activity given its ability to support relationships through musical interaction, in addition to being enjoyed in its own right by both those living with dementia and their carers.

Music has the ability to reach deep into the heart and mind of every individual. It can carry texts and emotions to a different level. It is a physical as well as a mental activity. Using the voice enables one of our most primal needs – the need to communicate with others of our species.

Deciding how to use music

As with choosing music for any act of worship, it is important to bear in mind a number of factors including the occasion, likely congregation (including questions of age and familiarity with the church), theme, and 'seasonal' influences. However, when considering hymns and songs that may be particularly appropriate for those living with dementia, additional elements come into play.

The planning required to hold a service in church will be different from that needed to take worship to a local residential home or day-care centre. In church you may be able to include two or three hymns within the context of a slightly longer service. Away from church, it may be better to aim for just one hymn to be included within a short, less formal act of worship.

In either case, stick with a few regular, simple items of basic repertoire that can be repeated or rotated each time to build familiarity and confidence, adding perhaps one 'seasonal' item

---

2 See, for example, W. T. Wallace, 'Memory for music: effect of melody on recall of text', *Journal of Experimental Psychology: Learning, Memory, and Cognition* 20 (1994), pp. 1471–85; C. Haslam and M. Cook, 'Striking a chord with amnesic patients: evidence that song facilitates memory', *Neurocase* 8 (2002), pp. 453–65.

each time. Remember that although repetition may appear boring to some, for those with dementia it is a means of deep recall and is helpful.

Provide the words in large, clear print and sing slightly slower than normal to allow those who are still able to follow the printed words to keep up and join in (but not so slowly that people falter or give up). Bear in mind that different versions of the words exist, especially where hymns have been updated to make the language more inclusive: this is likely to be unhelpful to those who learned 'original' words at an early age. This is also true of tunes – often the more traditional tune is the most familiar, though contemporary tunes for familiar hymns such as 'At the name of Jesus' and 'O Jesus, I have promised' have become largely ingrained in church repertoire. Be aware also that the pairing of words and tune can be a very localized phenomenon, and that very firm views are held as to what the 'right' tune should be!

Know your target group: are they, or have they been, largely regular members of your church family? If they are, then they will be familiar with your usual style of worship, hymns and songs, and you can choose music that will be likely to resonate with them. If there are people present whose familiar worship habits you don't know, consider whether it might be possible to ask them, or their carers or families, what experience they have of church. If this isn't possible, choose something that might be familiar from school. Also consider the overall age range of the group: it is no longer the case that post-Second World War secular songs are familiar – as the range of years in which the 'older generation' were born becomes more recent, you will need to look to the 1950s, 1960s and 1970s for inspiration in sourcing both church and secular music.

Encourage everyone to join in, even if they just want to hum along instead of singing the words, and consider providing a few percussion instruments for those who may no longer be able to sing at all.

If you are able to provide musical accompaniment, either on a keyboard or guitar, it will enable people to feel more secure in joining in, but bear in mind the guidance below on the range of the notes in the tune. Pre-recorded backing tracks are less suitable as they do not take either pitch or speed into consideration and may overwhelm rather than assist. If no instrumental accompaniment is available, a confident singer who is able to maintain accurate pitch and engage with the gathered community can also lead effectively.

At a technical musical level, it is worth bearing in mind that vocal range is narrower at both ends of the age spectrum: just as very young children have a limited range that gradually increases as they mature, so there then begins a steady decline in available notes as a person enters their seventies and beyond – particularly in those who have not sung regularly through adulthood.

The following principles are a good basic guide in choosing suitable repertoire, but the individual situation may override some or all of these on any occasion:[3]

- A range within the octave B-B works best for older voices – both male and female, especially when centred around F or G, though occasional rises to C or D are manageable provided there is not too much of a jump.
- Melodies that are modal rather than tonal, including plainsong, are easier to sing.
- Melodies that are strong without harmony (i.e. often few accidentals).
- Melodies that move largely by step, or with a few simple jumps: major/minor third, perfect fourth, perfect fifth, occasional major sixth (e.g. the hymn tune 'Crimond').
- Melodies with a regular metre that are mostly free of complex rhythmic patterns. Avoid if possible those that have

---

3 See P. E. Lynch, 'A liturgical repertory for small churches within the Scottish Episcopal Church', MA Dissertation, Music (Sacred Music Pathway), University of Bangor, 2010. Other principles from a presentation by Andrew Reid, then Director of the Royal School of Church Music, to the Diocesan Liturgical Advisers' conference on 'Accessible worship for those living with dementia', Church House, Westminster, 6 April 2017.

indeterminate rests mid-way (e.g. 'I, the Lord of sea and sky').

- Lutheran Chorales, Calvinist Psalm melodies and music from other liturgical traditions.
- Hymns and songs designed for unison singing (whether with or without accompaniment, unless the accompaniment is essential).
- Hymns sung by sports crowds ('Abide with me'; 'Guide me, O thou great Redeemer/ Jehovah') and at major national events (e.g. Remembrance Sunday).
- Hymns and songs familiar from school assembly and Sunday school.
- Tunes derived from folk sources: Celtic and other UK folk sources, from elsewhere around the world, carols.
- A simplified chordal accompaniment is sometimes easier for inexperienced singers to follow (and may give a less proficient accompanist the confidence to enjoy the experience).

A selection of hymns and songs is given below,[4] but there are many other possibilities:

Abba, Father, let me be
Abide with me
All people that on earth do dwell (Old Hundredth)
All things bright and beautiful
Alleluia, sing to Jesus
Amazing grace
And can it be that I should gain
And did those feet (Jerusalem)
Angel voices, ever singing
At the name of Jesus
Be still, for the presence of the Lord
Be thou my vision
Colours of day dawn into the mind

---

4 From a presentation by Andrew Reid, Director of the Royal School of Church Music, to the Diocesan Liturgical Advisers' conference on 'Accessible worship for those living with dementia', Church House, Westminster, 6 April 2017.

Come down, O Love divine
Dear Lord and Father of mankind
Eternal Father, strong to save
Father, hear the prayer we offer
Father, we love you, we worship and adore you
Fight the good fight
Firmly I believe, and truly
For all the saints
Give me joy in my heart/oil in my lamp (Sing hosanna)
Glory to thee, my God, this night
God forgave my sin in Jesus' name (freely, freely)
Great is thy faithfulness
Guide me, O thou great Redeemer
He who would valiant be
How lovely on the mountains (our God reigns)
I vow to thee, my country
Jesus, good above all other
Jesus shall reign, where'er the sun
Lead us, heavenly Father, lead us
Lord of all hopefulness, Lord of all joy
Love divine, all loves excelling
Loving shepherd of thy sheep
Make me a channel of your peace
Morning has broken
Now thank we all our God
O God, our help in ages past
O Jesus, I have promised
O Lord my God, when I in awesome wonder (How great
    thou art)
On a hill far away (The old rugged cross)
One more step along the world I go
Onward, Christian soldiers
Praise, my soul, the King of heaven
Praise to the holiest in the height
Rock of ages, cleft for me
Soul of my Saviour
Stand up, stand up for Jesus
Sweet Sacrament divine

Take my life and let it be
Tell out, my soul
The Church's one foundation
The day thou gavest
The Lord's my shepherd, I'll not want
There is a green hill far away
Thine be the glory
To God be the glory
We plough the fields and scatter
What a friend we have in Jesus
When I survey the wondrous cross

Afterword

SAM WELLS

The Baptist wasn't completely convinced about Jesus. 'Are you the one who is to come, or are we to wait for another?' Jesus had a simple answer: 'The blind receive their sight, the lame walk, the lepers are cleansed, the deaf hear, the dead are raised, the poor have good news brought to them.'

At my church we're won over by the rhetoric but a bit chary about the details. We're not sure about the blind receiving their sight: we focus on how people with visual impairment develop extraordinary depth of insight in other ways. Likewise, with the deaf: we're keen to focus on a person's assets rather than define them by their deficits. We'd probably make an exception for raising the dead – where the pastoral needs justified it, of course. We're all for upholding the poor, but we'd be anxious to hear what the poor had to say for themselves before assuming the only good news in their lives was the news that came from us.

But in spite of our inhibitions, we still see miracles. We still see the Holy Spirit do unbelievable things.

It is hard to categorize Alzheimer's. Once you've developed your scheme, in which there's disability, which you seek to live with, think beyond, understand, even befriend, and illness, which you seek to overcome, withstand, and not be defined by, then you have to work out in which category to put Alzheimer's. And you'd better decide pretty quickly because Alzheimer's is fast taking over. It hides itself away because those with the condition become less likely to enter public spaces. For that reason it's almost an invisible condition.

When I came to the church one woman stood out. You couldn't miss her. She would shout up from the congregation at unexpected moments. If you quoted Ecclesiasticus and said 'Let us now praise famous men', you wouldn't get as far as 'and our fathers that begat us' without her shouting up, 'And what about the women?' It was like a tripwire. If the role of preacher and presider one Sunday were both taken by men, you could be sure that as you greeted her at the door she would look at you with her withering gaze and say, 'Have you forgotten about the women?' There was no use arguing about taking turns and cherishing the gifts of all. She was a single-issue fanatic.

Although it wasn't just one issue. She had the same seek-and-destroy guided-missile approach when it came to vegetarianism. Rare was the clergy member who had not been cornered by her strong handshake, pleading escape from her vice-like grip as she 'talked and explained the Scriptures' as far as they made the consumption of meat unconscionable. From everything I was told, dementia hadn't made her a vigilante: she'd always been like that. If anything, her faltering faculties slightly reduced her passionate advocacy and scaled the volume down just a little.

She came to the first two evenings we organized around the topics of Dementia and Faith. She listened as people spoke movingly about caring for a beloved husband or mother and absorbingly about how dementia works and how its varieties differ. But then she made it clear she believed we could do better. She buttonholed two friends and hatched a plan. Over two lunches together they spoke and the two friends wrote things down, about her, about her life, about her mother, about her condition.

And so it was that we beheld her glory. On the third Dementia evening, she stood behind a lectern. In her hands were four pages of notes, typed out by her two friends from their conversations. And then she began to speak. Slowly, and with extraordinary dignity, she told us her story. And what a story. 'Mummy was Baroness von Hundelshausen. She spoke six languages. I was born in Mexico and brought to Britain as a baby.' She went on to speak of the 'battle': 'Jesus made it very clear that women are equal and not to be pushed around by men. But women's role in life and society has always been undervalued and must be equalized.'

She went on to speak of working for a newspaper and taking it over a few years later. 'It was really lovely because I could say anything I wanted to say.' She talked of being elected as a councillor for Westminster, and making sure that Buckingham Palace paid local taxes – which it had never done before. She talked of being radicalized by her mother's dementia, and realizing 'the Government didn't give a damn about old women'. But then, astonishingly, she spoke about her own experience of Alzheimer's. 'Fear and anger can be very close together, especially when you have memory problems, and I was angry.' She explained what we'd all experienced of being with her. 'I hate people deciding for me or speaking for me. I want people to understand that I'm still me, I still have a sense of self and my own rights.'

How awesome is the sight. Here was the one brought to Jesus through the roof by friends carrying a stretcher – through the roof of ignorance, prejudice, impatience and hasty judgement. And in that moment I saw what prophetic ministry means. Not berating authorities, not denouncing congregations, not excoriating government; but slowly, patiently, building sufficient trust with a person who is socially excluded, not assuming that one has to speak on their behalf, but over a transformative meal, listening, taking notes, assembling thoughts, so that one day, with a fair wind and a sympathetic audience, that person could speak her own words, sing her true song, and let the whole room thud with the sound of jaws dropping.

They that wait upon the Lord shall mount up with wings like eagles. That night I saw a miracle. I saw what the Church can be.

Summary of Advice and Recommendations

Chapter 1

Be alert to different patterns of behaviour for which allowance
  needs to be made.
Using all our senses gives a richer experience to worship and
  aids participation.
Sensory prompts can help access long-term memories.
Repetition and familiarity stimulate engagement.
Good eye contact is important, as is the use of direct, clear
  language.
Periods of quiet for reflection are important.
Involve carers in the planning of worship if at all possible.

Chapter 2

Dementia is as much a social as a medical condition.
People newly diagnosed with dementia are vulnerable to feelings of low self-worth and clinical depression.
In the more advanced phases of dementia, the ability to be
  mentally and physically still, to meditate and pray, may be
  lost.
A dementia-friendly community is more friendly to all.

Chapter 3

We all engage differently with worship.

Ritual can help in making services meaningful.

If practical, encourage members of the congregation to attend worship in the care home or hospital.

Chapter 4

Those who come to worship need to feel settled and safe.

Music and visual prompts can give clues and set the tone of what is about to happen.

Using older versions of Scripture and prayer books may be useful.

Use a variety of ways of engaging – such as group discussion, singing, craft, movement and dance, prayer activities.

Following a regular pattern of worship. Use simple liturgies and direct language.

Engage all the senses to make connections and spark interest and understanding.

Allow people with dementia to continue to minister to those around them, to the best of their ability.

Hold the service in church (if accessible).

Use simple ideas but show respect for the age and experience of the congregation.

Choose themes that have a clear link to the Christian message.

Consider the timing of the service: people living with dementia may struggle with an early start.

Keep the gathering fairly small so it doesn't become over-whelming.

A team of volunteers makes the process easier.

Offer tea and cake!

Chapter 5

Designate a member of the church to lead on dementia matters. Include their contact details in parish notices.

Immediate practicalities such as toilets, heating, lighting and sound amplification are important – but also think about the safety of the church building (especially flooring) and surrounding grounds.

A church can have a part to play in making the wider local community dementia-friendly.

Offer occasional memory-friendly services.

Remember the spiritual needs of the carer.

Offer to help with transport, or to arrange it.

Be mindful of 'prayers for healing' and what they might (inadvertently) suggest.

Not everyone with dementia has the support of a carer.

Be aware of the ongoing needs of those who were carers whose loved ones have passed away.

Chapter 6

Music improves emotional wellbeing.

Music can unlock texts and emotions.

Stick with a few regular, simple items that can be repeated or rotated.

For those with dementia, repetition is a means of deep recall.

Provide the words in large, clear print.

Use the traditional version of hymn words if they have been more recently modernized.

Use traditional tunes or those that have become familiar through school assembly, Sunday school, 'national' occasions, etc.

Look beyond the post-Second World War secular music to the 1950s, 1960s and 1970s for inspiration.

Encourage everyone to join in, even if they just want to hum.

Offer percussion instruments as an alternative to singing.

A simple accompaniment will enable people to feel more secure in joining in.

Vocal range reduces with age: adapt the pitch of hymns accordingly.
Simpler tunes work best.

Afterword

Organize non-worship events around dementia and faith.
Take time to build trust with a person who is socially excluded.
Do not assume a person with dementia is unable to speak on his or her own behalf.

Further Reading, Websites, and Bibliography for Individual Chapters

Further reading

Adams, T., *Developing Dementia-friendly Churches*, Cambridge: Grove Booklet P153.

Behers, R., *Spiritual Care for People Living with Dementia Using Multisensory Interventions: A Guide for Chaplains*, London: Jessica Kingsley Publishers, 2018.

Bryden, C., *Who Will I Be When I Die?*, London: Jessica Kingsley Publishers, 1998.

Bryden, C., *Dancing with Dementia*, London: Jessica Kingsley Publishers, 2005.

Coghlan, P., *Creating 'Church' at Home for Older People Living with Dementia*, Buxhall: Kevin Mayhew, 2016.

Collicutt, J., *Thinking of You: A Theological and Practical Resource for People Affected by Dementia*, Oxford: Bible Reading Fellowship, 2016.

Cooper, J., *Body, Soul, and Life Everlasting*, Grand Rapids, MI: Eerdmans, 1989.

Earey, M., *Worship that Cares*, London: SCM Press, 2012.

George, C., *Living Liturgies: Transition Time Resources for Services, Prayer and Conversation with Older People*, Oxford: Bible Reading Fellowship, 2015.

Goldsmith, M., *In a Strange Land . . . People with Dementia and the Local Church*, Southwell: 4M Publications, 2004.

Green, J., *What About the Soul? Neuroscience and Christian Anthropology*, Nashville, TN: Abingdon Press, 2004.

Jeeves, M., *Minds, Brains, Souls and Gods*, Leicester: Inter-Varsity Press, 2013.

MacKinlay, E. and Trevitt, C., *Facilitating Spiritual Reminiscence for People with Dementia: A Learning Guide*, London: Jessica Kingsley Publishers, 2015.

Morris, S., *Memory Café: How to Engage with Memory Loss and Build Community*, Cambridge: Grove Booklet MEv120.

Morse, L., *Dementia: Pathways to Hope: Spiritual Insights and Practical Advice*, Oxford: Lion Hudson, 2015.

Pickering, S., *Creative Ideas for Ministry with the Aged: Liturgies, Prayers and Resources*, Norwich: Canterbury Press, 2014.

Ramsey, J. L., *Dignity and Grace: Wisdom for Caregivers and those Living with Dementia*, Minneapolis, MN: Fortress Press, 2018.

Sampson, F., *Prayers for Dementia and How to Live Well with It*, London: Darton, Longman and Todd, 2017.

Saunders, J., *Dementia: Pastoral Theology and Pastoral Care*, Cambridge: Grove Booklet P89.

Woodward, J., *Between Remembering and Forgetting: The Spiritual Dimensions of Dementia*, London: Continuum, 2010.

Woodward, J. and Carr, W., *Valuing Age: Pastoral Ministry with Older People*, London: SPCK, 2008.

Websites

www.godlyplay.uk/method/
www.storiesforthesoul.org
www.thegiftofyears.org.uk/messy-vintage
www.messychurch.org.uk
www.carersfirst.org.uk/
https://godlyplaymutualblessings.wordpress.com/deep-talk/
www.messychurch.org.uk/messyvintage
www.annachaplaincy.org.uk/
https://livability.org.uk/
www.ageuk.org.uk/
www.alzheimers.org.uk/
www.differentbrains.org/resources/alzheimers/
www.dementiauk.org/
www.mha.org.uk/

Bibliography for individual chapters

Chapter 1

Augustine, *Confessions*, trans. Henry Chadwick, Oxford: Oxford University Press, 1991, pp. 186–7.

Chittister, J., *The Gift of Years*, London: Darton, Longman and Todd, 2008.

Teilhard de Chardin, P., *Le Milieu Divin*, Paris, 1957; English translation, London: Collins & Sons, 1960.

Chapter 2

Augustine, *Confessions*, trans. Henry Chadwick, Oxford: Oxford University Press, 1991.

Batson, C. D., Schoenrade, P. and Ventis, W. L., *Religion and the Individual: A Social-Psychological Perspective*, New York: Oxford University Press, 1993.

Baumeister, R., *Meanings of Life*, New York: Guilford, 1992.

Berryman, J., *Godly Play: An Imaginative Approach to Religious Education*, San Francisco, CA: Harper, 1991.

Cavalletti, S., *The Religious Potential of the Child*, Chicago, IL: Archdiocese of Chicago, 1993.

Coles, A., 'The discipline of neurology', in A. Coles and J. Collicutt (eds), *Neurology and Religion*, Cambridge: Cambridge University Press, 2019.

Collicutt, J., 'Posttraumatic growth, spirituality, and acquired brain injury', *Brain Impairment* 12 (2011a), pp. 82–92.

Collicutt, J., 'Psychology, religion and spirituality', *The Psychologist* 24 (2011b), pp. 250–1.

Collicutt, J., *Thinking of You: A Theological and Practical Resource for People Affected by Dementia*, Oxford: Bible Reading Fellowship, 2016.

Collicutt, J., *When You Pray: Daily Bible Reflections on the Lord's Prayer*, Oxford: Bible Reading Fellowship, 2019.

Cooper, J., *Body, Soul, and Life Everlasting*, Grand Rapids, MI: Eerdmans, 1989.

Earey, M., *Worship that Cares*, London: SCM Press, 2012.

Feil, N., *The Validation Breakthrough: Simple Techniques for Communicating with People with Alzheimer's and Other Dementias*, Baltimore, MD: Health Professions Press, 2002.

Goldsmith, M., *In a Strange Land . . .: People with Dementia and the Local Church*, Southwell: 4M Publications, 2004.

Gomes, P., *The Good Book: Reading the Bible with Mind and Heart*, New York: Harper, 2002.

Green, J., *What About the Soul? Neuroscience and Christian Anthropology*, Nashville, TN: Abingdon Press, 2004.

Hands, I., 'Liturgy is an anchor – don't brush it aside', *Church Times*, 3 May 2019, www.churchtimes.co.uk/articles/2019/3-may/comment/opinion/liturgy-is-an-anchor-don-t-brush-it-aside.

Huguelet, P. and Koenig, H., 'Introduction: key concepts', in P. Huguelet and H. Koenig (eds), *Religion and Spirituality in Psychiatry*, Cambridge: Cambridge University Press, 2009, pp. 1–5.

Jeeves, M., *Minds, Brains, Souls and Gods*, Leicester: Inter-Varsity Press, 2013.

Kitwood, T., *Dementia Reconsidered: The Person Comes First*, Maidenhead: Open University Press, 1997.

Pargament, K., 'Religious methods of coping: sources for the conservation and transformation of significance', in E. Shafranske (ed.), *Religion and the Clinical Practice of Psychology*, Washington, DC: American Psychological Association, 1996, pp. 215–35.

Pargament, K., *The Psychology of Religion and Coping*, New York: Guilford, 2001.

Pembroke, N., *Pastoral Care in Worship: Liturgy and Psychology in Dialogue*, London: T&T Clark, 2009.

Saver, J. and Rabin, J., 'The neural substrates of religious experience', *Journal of Neuropsychiatry and Clinical Neuroscience* 9 (1997), pp. 498–510.

Slater, V. and Collicutt, J., 'Living Well in the End Times (LWET): a project to research and support churches' engagement with issues of death and dying', *Practical Theology* 11 (2018), pp. 176–88.

Smith, S. M., *Caring Liturgies: The Pastoral Power of Christian Ritual*, Minneapolis, MN: Fortress Press, 2012.

Sorrell, J., 'Listening in thin places: ethics in the care of persons with Alzheimer's disease', *Advances in Nursing Science* 29 (2006), pp. 152–60.

Swinton, J., *Dementia: Living in the Memories of God*, London: SCM Press, 2012.

Warner, M., 'Incarnation and church growth', in D. Goodhew (ed.), *Towards a Theology of Church Growth*, London: Routledge, 2015, pp. 107–26.

Watts, F., *Theology and Psychology*, Aldershot: Ashgate, 2002.

Welsh, P., 'Time to retreat from throw-away liturgy', *Church Times*, 15 June 2018, www.churchtimes.co.uk/articles/2018/15-june/comment/opinion/time-to-retreat-from-throwaway-liturgy.

Willard, D., *The Spirit of the Disciplines: Understanding how God Changes Lives*, New York: HarperCollins, 1988.

Williams, R., *Resurrection: Interpreting the Easter Gospel*, London: Darton, Longman and Todd, 2014.

Chapter 3

Archbishops' Council, *Transforming Worship: Living the New Creation. A Report by the Liturgical Commission* (GS 1651), London: Archbishops' Council, 2007.

Austin, J. L., *How to Do Things with Words*, Oxford: Clarendon Press, 1962.

Barton, J. and Muddiman, J. (eds), *Oxford Bible Commentary*, Oxford, Oxford University Press, 2007.

Bryden, C., 'Letter to the Church', *Journal of Disability and Religion* 22 (2018), pp. 96–106.

Eldred, J. B. et al., 'Your heart can dance to them even if your feet can't', *Practical Theology* 7 (2014), pp. 153–79.

Goldsmith, M., 'When words are no longer necessary: the gift of ritual', *Journal of Religious Gerontology* 12 (2002), 139–50.

Goodall, M. A., 'The evaluation of spiritual care in a dementia care setting', *Dementia* 8 (2009), pp. 167–83.

Higgins, P., '"It's a consolation": the role of Christian religion for people with dementia who are living in care homes', *Journal of Religion, Spirituality and Aging* 26 (2014), pp. 320–29.

Keck, D., *Forgetting Whose We Are: Alzheimer's Disease and the Love of God*, Nashville, TN: Abingdon Press, 1996.

Kennedy, E. et al., 'Christian worship leaders' attitudes and observations of people with dementia', *Dementia* 13 (2014), pp. 586–97.

Kevern, P., 'The grace of foolishness: what Christians with dementia can bring to the churches', *Practical Theology* 2 (2009), pp. 205–18.

Kevern, P., '"I pray that I will not fall over the edge": what is left of faith after dementia?', *Practical Theology* 4 (2011), pp. 283–94.

Marcus, J., *Mark 8—16: A New Translation with Introduction and Commentary*, New Haven, CT: Yale University Press, 2009.

Phinney, A., 'Horizons of meaning in dementia: retained and shifting narratives', *Journal of Religion, Spirituality and Aging* 23 (2011), pp. 254–68.

Russell, M., 'Listening to dementia: a new paradigm for theology?', *Contact* 135 (2001), pp. 13–21.

Suggs, P. K. and Suggs, Douglas L., 'The understanding and creation of rituals: enhancing the life of older adults', *Journal of Religious Gerontology* 15 (2003), pp. 17–24.

Swinton, J., 'Building a Church for strangers', *Journal of Religion, Disability and Health* 4 (2001), pp. 25–63.

Underwood, R., 'Alzheimer's', available from www.richard-underwood.com. © Richard Underwood. Used by permission.

Vaught, L., 'Worship models and music in spiritual formation', *Journal of Religion, Spirituality and Aging* 22 (2009), pp. 104–19.

Chapter 4

All Party Parliamentary Group on Arts, Health and Wellbeing, *Creative Health: The Arts for Health and Wellbeing*, 2017.

Bamford, S. M. and Bowell, S., 'What would life be – without a song or a dance, what are we?', *A Report from the Commission on Dementia and Music, International Longevity Centre*, 2018.

Berryman, J. W., *Teaching Godly Play: How to Mentor the Spiritual Development of Children*, New York: Morehouse Education Resources, 2009.

George, C., *Living Liturgies: Transition Time Resources for Services, Prayer and Conversation with Older People*, Oxford: Bible Reading Fellowship, 2015.

Howard, L. W., *Using Godly Play with Alzheimer's and Dementia Patients*, New York: Morehouse Education Resources, 2015. Available at: www.churchpublishing.org/products/usinggodlyplay withalzheimersanddementiapatients.

Steinhauser, M. and Oystese, R., *Godly Play: European Perspectives on Practice and Research*, Münster: Waxmann, 2018.

Vella-Burrows, T., *Singing and People with Dementia*, Sidney De Haan Research Centre for Arts and Health, 2012.

Chapter 5

'Illness and independence', *The Times*, 28 December 2017, available from https://www.thetimes.co.uk/article/illness-and-independence-50h9wzb5x.

Chapter 6

Haslam, C. and Cook, M., 'Striking a chord with amnesic patients: evidence that song facilitates memory', *Neurocase* 8 (2002), pp. 453–65.

Lynch, P. E., 'A liturgical repertory for small churches within the Scottish Episcopal Church', MA Dissertation, Music (Sacred Music Pathway), University of Bangor, 2010.

Verghese, J., Lipton, R. B., Katz, M. J., Hall, C. B., Derby, C. A., Kuslansky, G., 'Leisure activities and the risk of dementia in the elderly', *The New England Journal of Medicine* 348 (2003), pp. 2508–16.

Wallace, W. T., 'Memory for music: effect of melody on recall of text', *Journal of Experimental Psychology: Learning, Memory, and Cognition* 20 (1994), pp. 1471–85.

Other principles from a presentation by Andrew Reid, then Director of the Royal School of Church Music, to the Diocesan Liturgical Advisers' conference on accessible worship for those living with dementia, Church House, Westminster, 6 April 2017.

Index

age:
and dementia 4, 11, 89, 102
and vocal range 114–15,
124
agency:
loss of 41, 88
and worship 48, 87
aggression 4
Alzheimer's disease 4, 14,
40, 66, 118, 120
and cognition 22
early stage 73
and internal logic 15
and loss of autonomy 88
and memory 16, 22, 26
treatment 89
Alzheimer's Society 91–2,
98–9, 108
Anderson, E. 86–7, 110
anxiety 5, 33, 61
Augustine of Hippo, St 7, 28
Austin, J. 46
autonomy *see* agency
awareness, spiritual 14,
16–36
and cognition 21–4, 25, 45
as homing instinct 20–1,
24, 28
and human spirit 16, 17–19

and role of worship 28–36

baptism, and Body of Christ
53, 54
behaviour:
changes in 4, 16, 25, 52,
88, 99, 121
responses to 40
unusual 49, 55–6, 68–9
Berryman, J. 29, 70
Body of Christ, Church as 5,
31, 37–8, 41, 50
Boisen, A. 50–1
Book of Common Prayer 32,
34–6, 98
Bryden, C. 37, 48–9, 51–2,
58–9
Burton-Jones, J. 29, 99

care homes:
and Godly Play 72–7, 78
and Messy Vintage 82–3
worship in 58, 96, 101,
112, 122
care staff, and Godly Play
79–80
carers:
and cost of caring 11–12,
86

with dementia 2–3
and guilt 3
respecting 108
and shared stories 41
support for 96, 98, 101,
106–8
and worship 5–6, 68, 86–7,
123
Cavalletti, S. 29
Celebration, in Messy
Vintage 81, 84–5
children, and people with
dementia 73
Chittister, J. 12
Church as Body of Christ 5,
31, 37–8, 41, 50
and diversity 44, 53, 56
learning from people with
dementia 52–9
and spiritual communion 52
and worship 54
churches, ageing
congregations 1, 80–1
churches, dementia-friendly
1, 65–6, 86–110, 123
and carers 106–8, 123
challenges for 86, 87–9, 99,
102–6
and commitment 108–10
Enabler 87, 90–4, 97
listening to people with
dementia 98–100, 109
marks of 86–7
and pastoral care 95–6, 101
and physical barriers to
inclusion 95
and services in care homes
96, 122

social activities 100
Churches Together in
Cumbria 90–1
clinical pastoral movement
51
cognition:
and learning difficulties 40
and personhood 8, 43, 48
and spiritual awareness
21–4, 25, 45
and worship 2, 43, 49, 52,
60–1, 101
Collicut, J. 25, 42
Common Worship 50
communication:
difficulties 15, 50, 62, 87,
94
and music 112
non-verbal 31, 71
community:
building 72–7
dementia-friendly 36, 96,
98, 110, 121, 123
and isolation 15, 98, 100
and personhood 8–9, 23–4,
34, 51, 55
concentration, loss of 4,
60–1, 63, 101
confusion 5, 6–7, 13, 87, 94,
110
congregations, ageing 1,
80–1
craft work, and worship 63,
64, 71, 81, 83–4
creativity:
and Godly Play 71
and Messy Church 63–4,
81, 83–4

dance, in worship 64
Davis, R. 58
Deep Talk 79–80
dementia:
  and age 4, 11, 89, 102
  cost 89
  diagnosing 4, 99
  early stages 5, 10, 39, 44
  early-onset 44, 66, 89, 94
  fear of 1–3, 5, 8, 120
  forms see Alzheimer's
    disease; dementia
    with Lewy bodies;
    frontotemporal dementia;
    vascular dementia
  numbers affected 89
  positive gains 24–8
  range of symptoms 39–40
  research 89, 99, 102,
    109–10
  search for a cure 33, 99,
    104–5, 109
  as social condition 15, 16,
    22–4, 118–19, 121
  and stigma 88
  and support services 91, 92,
    96, 102
  symptoms 4–5, 60
  treatment 89, 99
  see also worship
dementia cafés 72
Dementia Enablers 87, 90–4,
  97
Dementia Friends 65, 91–2,
  97, 99
dementia with Lewy bodies
  4, 88
depression 5, 22–3, 33, 121

Descartes, René 6, 18
dignity, human 1–2, 43, 56
disease, and dementia 39–40
diversity, and Body of
  Christ 44, 53, 56

Earey, M. 33
Eldred, J. B. 51
emotions:
  expression 44
  and faith 10
  and meaning-making 24–5,
    27
  and music 112, 123
empathy, and relationships
  16, 21, 23, 101–2
Eucharist:
  and Body of Christ 53, 56
  and cognition 43
  and Godly Play 29
  and re-membering 30–3, 36
executive function, impaired
  22, 23, 26
experiences, shared 38,
  39–44, 63, 84
eye contact 10, 121

faith:
  dementia as challenge to
    103–5
  and feelings 10, 44, 101
  and prayer 57–8
  sustaining 101
familiarity, in worship 10,
  63, 112, 121
Feast, in Godly Play 29, 71,
  77, 78, 80
friendship, need for 5, 51,
  88, 100, 101

frontotemporal dementia 4, 88
and executive function 22, 26

George, C. 67
Godly Play 28–9, 64, 69–72
and building of community 72–7
challenges of 78–80
Feast 29, 71, 77, 78, 80
and mental and spiritual health 75–6
and reminiscence 73–4
Response Time 67–8, 71, 74, 75, 76–7
and wondering 70–2, 73–4
see also Messy Vintage
Goldsmith, M. 46–7
Grace, The 85
Guardini, R. 53
guilt, of carers 3

Hauerwas, Stanley 43
healing, prayer for 105, 109, 123
Higgins, P. 43, 45
holding cross 9
holy fool figure 55–6
Holy Spirit:
and Body of Christ 54
and human spirit 17–19, 28
and prayer 9–10
homing instinct 20–1, 24, 28
hope, and memory 23, 32
hospital, worship in 58, 112
Howard, L. W. 71–2
humour 106

Hunt, William Holman, *The Awakening Conscience* 21
hymns:
and accompaniment 113–14, 115, 123
familiar 11, 51, 62, 67, 85, 98, 112–13, 123
suggested 115–17
and tunes 113–15, 123
and vocal range 114–15, 124

identity, and memory 22
image of God 5, 8, 16, 21, 39, 41
imagery:
of sheep and shepherd 54
visual 9
implicational system 25–6
inclusion:
barriers to 85, 98, 99
in worship 5, 86
individuals, respecting 72–7, 87, 99, 122
inhibition, loss of 27
introversion 5
isolation 5, 15, 98, 100

Keck, D. 41
Kevern, P. 40, 43, 55

lament, healthy 33
language, and cognition 22, 25, 60–1
learning difficulties, and cognition 40
Leontius of Neapolis, *Life of Symeon the Holy Fool* 55

Liturgical Commission
(Church of England) 53
Liturgical Movement 48
liturgy, renewal 49, 53–4, 61
see also Godly Play; Messy
Vintage; worship
Livability 78, 94
logic, internal 15
Lord's Prayer 27, 46, 52
traditional words 10, 32,
36, 62, 68, 85

Marcus, J. 57
meaning-making 21, 22, 45,
51–2
in accessible worship 63
and emotions 24–5, 27
in Godly Play 71, 75–6
and habitus 27–8, 35
memory:
in Alzheimer's disease 14,
16, 22, 26
bodily 32
explicit 26
and identity 22
long-term 11, 61, 62, 84,
85, 98, 121
painful 12–13
and personhood 2, 6–8,
8–9
and senses 9, 26, 64, 74,
121
short-term 61, 62
and worship 2, 50–1, 62,
67
Messy Church 81–3
Messy Vintage 64, 80–5
and The Grace 85

see also Godly Play
ministry:
by people with dementia
64, 77, 122
to the elderly 95–6, 101,
102–3
Montessori, Maria 70
movement, in worship 61,
64
music 111–20, 122
effects 50–1, 63, 85, 97
and memory 10–11, 61,
111–12
and wellbeing 111, 123

noise, as confusing 10

othering, of people with
dementia 39
over-stimulation, in worship
61

Pargament, K. 35
participation in worship 38,
45–52, 63, 68–9, 71–9
and vocalization 48–50, 62
Pembroke, N. 30
personality change 14, 88
personhood:
and community 8–9, 23–4,
34, 52, 55
and memory 2, 6–8, 8–9
and rationality 6, 8, 43, 48
Phinney, A. 45
pneuma (spirit) 17–18,
19–20
population, ageing 1, 4, 11
prayer:
familiar 46, 61, 62

for healing 105
with holding cross 9
and memory 27–8, 85
for people with dementia
57, 100, 109–10
of reminiscence 7, 9
psuche:
and cognition 21, 26–7, 33
and *sōma* 18–19
and worship 31–2
rationality:
and cognition 22, 25, 44,
49
and internal logic 15
and personhood 6, 8, 43
reflection, in worship 10,
75, 85
relationships, and empathy
16, 21, 23, 101–2
reminiscence, in worship 7,
9, 63, 73–4
repetition, in worship 10,
112–13, 121, 123
Response Time, in Godly
Play 67–8, 71, 74, 75,
76–7
restlessness 4
resurrection, and the body
19
ritual, value 46–8, 122
Russell, M. 44

sacraments *see* baptism;
Eucharist
Sacrosanctum Concilium 49
sarx (flesh) 17–18, 19–20
Scripture, older versions 10,
62, 98, 122

Second Vatican Council, and
liturgy 48, 49, 53
self-awareness 51–2, 120
loss 16
self-worth 21, 22–3, 76–7,
121
senses:
and memory 9, 26, 74, 121
in worship 9, 10–11, 61,
64, 78, 121–2
silence, in worship 61, 63
singing, effects 63, 112, 113
Smith, S. M. 34
sōma, and *psuche* 18–19
songs from childhood 11,
61, 62, 111–12
stories:
in Godly Play 70–1
listening to 39–44
in worship 64
Stories for the Soul 64, 69,
78, 79, 80
Suggs, P. 47
Swinton, John 28, 40, 41,
43–4, 54, 56–7

Tea Services 97
Teilhard de Chardin, P. 13
Teresa of Avila, St 109
theology, and shared
experiences 38, 39–44
training:
for Enablers 97
for Godly Play 79
transcendence deficits 21

Underhill, Evelyn 12
Underwood, R., 'Alzheimer's'
42

vascular dementia 4, 88
  and cognition 22, 26
  and memory 26
Vaught, L. 48
visual-spatial awareness 4–5

Watts, F. 25
weakness, and Body of Christ
  9, 19, 52–6, 59
Wellbeing boxes 74, 74
Welsh, P. 35
Willard, D. 18
Williams, R. 23
wondering, and Godly Play
  70–2, 73–4
worship 1–5
  and agency 48, 87
  and atmosphere 62
  in care home or hospital
  58–9, 72–7, 82, 96, 101,
  112, 122

and carers 5–6, 10
designing 9–11, 60–85
inclusive 5, 86
learning from people with
  dementia 52–9
and movement 61, 64
and music 112–17, 122
need for quiet reflection 10,
  75, 85, 95
and participation 38,
  45–52, 63, 68–9, 71–9
and quality of life 37
and senses 9, 37, 61, 64,
  74, 121, 122
and spiritual awareness
  28–36
themes 63–4, 67, 81, 83–5,
  97, 112, 122
theology of 37–59

Yeats, W. B., 'Lapis Lazuli' 3

BIBLICAL REFERENCES

Old Testament
Genesis
  1.26–31   5
  1.27   8

Leviticus
  19.14   86
  19.32   1

Isaiah
  49.15–16   9

Psalms
  22   34
  23   54
  71   vii
  71.17–18   37
  88   6, 33
  91.5–6   110

Ruth
  1.16   108

New Testament

Matthew
16.17	20
17	57
25.40	53, 59

Mark
4.26–29	83
9	57
10.15	27

John
3.3–4 27	
3.6–7	20
3.16	77
6.12 13	

Acts
| 17.25b–28 | 20 |

Romans
8.7–9a, 14	17
8.15b–16	18
8.26–27	9–10

1 Corinthians
3.16	54
10.17	53
12	5, 56
12.12	56
12.13	53
12.17	56
12.21	56
12.26	53
15.42–44	19

2 Corinthians
4.7–12	59
11.30	55
12.9b–10	55
13.4	55

Philippians
| 2.13 | 28 |

Colossians
| 3.1 | 20 |

Index created by Meg Davies